AF597972

Motor Neurons - New Insights

Edited by Natalia Szejko and Kamila Saramak

Published in London, United Kingdom

Motor Neurons - New Insights
http://dx.doi.org/10.5772/intechopen.110975
Edited by Natalia Szejko and Kamila Saramak

Contributors
Alec S.T. Smith, Changho Chun, David L. Mack, Jinmyoung Joo, Juyoung Seong, Kamila Saramak, Makiko Tani, Mudassar Nazar Khan, Natalia Szejko, Till Marquardt, Toshiaki Suzuki, Wendy Wenqiao Yang

First published in London, United Kingdom, 2024 by IntechOpen
IntechOpen is the global imprint of INTECHOPEN LIMITED, registered in England and Wales, registration number: 11086078, 167-169 Great Portland Street, London, W1W 5PF, United Kingdom

British Library Cataloguing-in-Publication Data
A catalogue record for this book is available from the British Library

Additional hard and PDF copies can be obtained from orders@intechopen.com

Motor Neurons - New Insights
Edited by Natalia Szejko and Kamila Saramak
p. cm.
Print ISBN 978-1-83768-966-8
Online ISBN 978-1-83768-967-5
eBook (PDF) ISBN 978-1-83768-968-2

Meet the editors

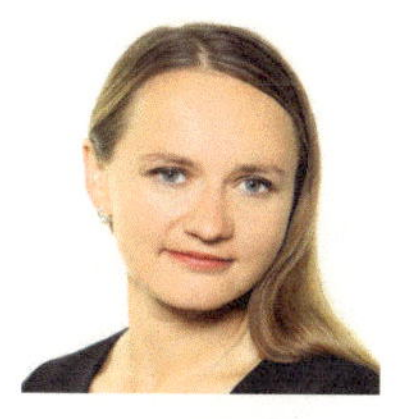

Natalia Szejko, MD, Ph.D., ScD, is a clinical and research fellow in the Department of Clinical Neurosciences, University of Calgary, Canada. She is also an assistant professor in the Department of Bioethics at the Medical University of Warsaw, Poland. She has completed her residency in the Department of Neurology at the Medical University of Warsaw. She also finished her Ph.D. in 2018 at the University of Warsaw and her ScD in 2020 at the Medical University of Warsaw. In 2020–2021 she held a postdoctoral fellowship at the Department of Neurology, Yale University, USA. She has complemented her education with a variety of clinical and research fellowships in Germany, Spain, Austria, and the USA. Her main areas of interest are movement disorders such as tics and neuroimmunology. She is secretary of the European Society for the Study of Tourette's Syndrome and co-author of the new European guidelines issued by this society, as well as an author of more than 50 publications and book chapters, mainly dedicated to movement disorders.

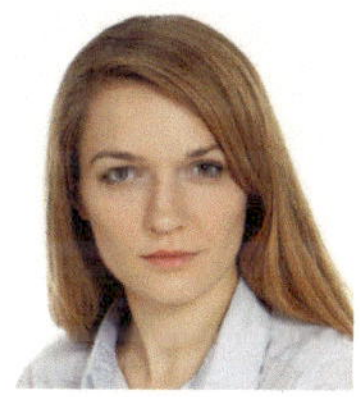

Kamila Saramak, MD, is a neurology resident in the Department of Neurology at the Hochzirl Hospital in Austria. She graduated from the Medical University of Warsaw in 2018. She completed her education with a variety of trainings organized by the German Neurological Society (DGN) as well as the American Academy of Neurology (AAN). Her main areas of interest are movement disorders and neuropharmacology. She is the author of several publications and book chapters, mainly dedicated to the use of cannabis-based medicine in neurological disorders.

Contents

Preface

Motor neuron diseases (MNDs) are a clinically and pathologically heterogenous group of neurodegenerative disorders, which are associated with progressive damage of the upper (UMN) or lower motor neurons (LMN) or both. MNDs encompass disorders such as amyotrophic lateral sclerosis (ALS), spinal muscular atrophy (SMA), spinobulbar muscular atrophy (SBMA), and hereditary spastic paraparesis (HSP). The involvement of the LMN manifests with muscle weakness, atrophy, and fasciculations. On the other hand, the degradation of the UMN leads to spastic paresis, hyperreflexia, clonus, and positive Babinski sign. Due to a wide variety of clinical phenotypes, complex genetical background, as well as the absence of reliable biomarkers, some MNDs still pose a diagnostic challenge for clinicians. Regarding SMA, the unraveling of the underlying genetical pathology led to the discovery of three efficacious and safe therapeutic interventions. These therapies, however, are not curative. Concerning ALS, the most common form of ALS has been identified in the course of intense research over 50 potentially causative or disease-modifying genes. Sadly, despite these advances, treatment options remain limited for the majority of ALS patients. In this book, we address the latest scientific updates in the genetics, pathophysiology, diagnostics, and treatment of MNDs.

Natalia Szejko
Department of Clinical Neurosciences,
University of Calgary,
Alberta, Canada

Department of Bioethics,
Medical University of Warsaw,
Warsaw, Poland

Kamila Saramak
Department of Neurology,
Hochzirl Hospital,
Zirl, Austria

Chapter 1

Introductory Chapter: Motor Neurons – New Insights

Kamila Saramak and Natalia Szejko

1. Introduction

Motor neuron diseases (MNDs) are a group of progressive neurodegenerative disorders associated with the degradation of the upper (UMN) and lower motor neurons (LMN), without affecting sensory and autonomic systems [1]. MNDs can be classified based on the pattern of motor neuron involvement; they encompass pure LMN syndromes, mixed upper and lower motor neuron diseases, and pure UMN syndromes [2]. MNDs patients display a large heterogeneity of clinical symptoms, including muscular weakness, atrophy, and corticospinal tract signs in varying combinations and severities, presenting a unique diagnostic challenge to clinicians [3]. In this chapter, we provide an overview of MNDs, in particular amyotrophic lateral sclerosis (ALS), spinal muscular atrophy (SMA), spinobulbar muscular atrophy (SBMA), and hereditary spastic paraparesis (HSP) [2].

2. Lower motor neuron (LMN) syndromes

The pure LMN syndromes are characterized by a selective degeneration of the anterior horn cells in the spinal cord and the motor nuclei in the brain stem, which inevitably leads to muscle weakness, atrophy, and fasciculations. They encompass spinal muscular atrophy (SMA) and spinobulbar muscular atrophy (SBMA), which is also known as Kennedy's disease [4]. Progressive muscular atrophy (PMA) will be described together with ALS [5].

2.1 Spinal muscular atrophy (SMA)

SMA is an autosomal recessive disease with a prevalence of 1 per 10,000 live born infants. It is most often related to mutations in the *Survival Motor Neuron 1 (SMN1)* gene, which encodes SMN, a protein essential for the development and survival of motor neurons. A paralogous gene, *SMN2*, also encodes the SMN protein but produces considerably less of it. SMA is associated with the degradation of anterior horn cells in the spinal cord and motor nuclei in the brain stem, producing weakness of limb, trunk, bulbar, and respiratory muscles [6]. SMA can be classified into five types (SMA 0–IV) according to age of onset and its clinical course. The beginning of symptoms varies from before birth (type 0) to adulthood (type IV) [7]. SMA type 0 is the rarest and the most severe form of SMA, usually resulting in death due to respiratory failure and bulbar deterioration within the first month of life. SMA type I is the most common form, accounting for approximately 60% of SMA cases, and, if not treated, leads to death by 2 years of age. The other SMA variants (II, III, and IV) are usually less debilitating [6].

The three relatively new therapies (nusinersen, onasemnogene abeparvovec, and risdiplam) have proven to be effective in slowing the progression of SMA. The first milestone has been reached with the discovery of nusinersen (marketed as Spinraza®), a modified antisense oligonucleotide drug that influences the splicing of the SMN2 pre-messenger RNA and thus enhances the expression of the full-length SMN protein. The intrathecal administration of nusinersen prolongs survival and significantly enhances the motor function both in pediatric and adult SMA patients [8, 9]. Onasemnogene abeparvovec (Zolgensma®) was the first single-dose gene-replacement SMA therapy approved in the USA and Europe [10]. The third drug, risdiplam (Evrysdi®), is a molecule that binds the SMN2 pre-mRNA in two locations, consequently increasing levels of the functional SMN protein. Risdiplam administered orally significantly increases survival and leads to motor improvement of patients with SMA compared with a natural history cohort [11, 12]. Numerous clinical trials and real-world data support the efficacy and safety profiles of the available drugs, which are meanwhile becoming new standards of therapy and may redefine the natural course of the disease. Nevertheless, there is still a number of important issues that need to be addressed, such as lack of evidence regarding superiority of one product compared to the others and combined therapies [13, 14].

In addition, stem cell-based treatments have shown the potential to repair the injured tissue and differentiate into neurons in animal models of SMA. Its therapeutic clinical translation, however, remains a challenge and requires further investigations [15, 16].

2.2 Spinobulbar muscular atrophy (SBMA)

SBMA is characterized by progressive weakness and atrophy of the proximal limb and bulbar muscles. The disease has its onset in adulthood, progresses much slower than other MNDs, and is X-linked. It is caused by a CAG repeat expansion in the androgen receptor gene and therefore affects exclusively males [17]. The life span of individuals with SBMA is typically normal; some patients, nonetheless, may be constrained to wheelchairs 15–20 years after symptom onset. Moreover, SMBA patients often show hormonal disturbances like gynecomastia, testicular atrophy, and reduced fertility [18]. Despite collaborative effort in developing therapeutic strategies, no curative treatment has been found up to this date. The latest preclinical studies focus on modifying the activity of androgen receptor (AR) in a selective manner [19].

3. Mixed upper and lower motor neuron diseases

3.1 Amyotrophic lateral sclerosis (ALS)

The term "motor neuron disease" encompasses, among others, amyotrophic lateral sclerosis (ALS), which with its prevalence of about 5.5–9.9 per 100,000 persons is the most frequent form of MND [20, 21]. ALS, also known as Lou Gehrig's disease, is believed to have a large genetic component; hence, its prevalence depends strongly on the study population, being higher in Australia, Europe, and North America, than in Asia [22]. The disease is more common in men than in women, especially in the younger groups of patients with ALS [23]. In most individuals with ALS, symptoms first appear in the sixth decade of life [24]. There are, however, other rare presentations of the disease. "Juvenile ALS," which is typically associated with a positive family history and slow progression, starts before 25 years of age, whereas the patients with sporadic "young-onset ALS" develop symptoms before reaching 45 years of age [25, 26].

In ALS, neuronal degeneration typically occurs in the cortex (UMN), as well as in the brain stem and the spinal cord (LMN) [27]. The majority of ALS patients present with limb onset of the disease, whereas bulbar onset of ALS occurs in up to 30% of the patients [28]. The disease progresses rapidly, spreading to various body regions, including respiratory muscles, causing death within 2–3 years for the bulbar onset cases and 3–5 years for the limb onset cases [27]. Recent studies regarding disease progression have led to a development of the model to predict survival without tracheostomy and noninvasive ventilation depending on a number of individual factors [29]. An overview of clinical spectrum of the most important ALS phenotypes is shown in **Table 1**.

The original diagnostic criteria for ALS were defined at El Escorial in 1990 and revised multiple times [30]. In 2019, the Gold Coast criteria were developed,

Phenotype	Affected motor neurons	Important features
Classical spinal onset (Charcot's type)	UMN + LMN	asymmetric weakness in a limb, which progresses to a contralateral limb or to other spinal and/or bulbar areas
Flail arm (Vulpian-Bernhardt's type)	LMN in UEs, UMN in LEs	predominantly proximal, progressive and symmetric wasting, and paresis of the upper limb muscles, while lower limbs and bulbar muscles are spared; occasionally present UMN signs in the legs
Flail leg (Marie-Patrikios' type, or a peroneal form of ALS)	LMN in LEs	asymmetric weakness confined to the lumbosacral spinal cord region that spreads to cervical and lumbar regions
Progressive bulbar palsy	LMN	the onset of dysarthria or dysphagia with bulbar muscle atrophy and fasciculations, with progression to the limbs
Pseudobulbar palsy	UMN	the onset of dysarthria or dysphagia with emotional lability with progression to the limbs, no bulbar muscle atrophy and no fasciculations
Progressive muscular atrophy	LMN	clinically isolated LMN syndrome typically starting in distal limb muscles in an asymmetric manner and spreading over months or years; some patients develop ALS with UMN signs
Primary lateral sclerosis	UMN	typically symmetrical onset with UMN signs in the lower limbs, many patients with PLS develop lower motor neuron signs within 4 years of symptom onset
Hemiplegic form	UMN	disease onset with unilateral UMN involvement, slow progression to the contralateral side; after a variable period evolution to ALS with LMN signs
Respiratory form	UMN + LMN	respiratory involvement followed by limb weakness

UMN: upper motor neuron; LMN: lower motor neuron; UE: upper extremity; LE: lower extremity; ALS: amyotrophic lateral sclerosis; and PLS: primary lateral sclerosis.

Table 1.
An overview of clinical spectrum of the most important ALS phenotypes.

increasing the diagnostic sensitivity for amyotrophic lateral sclerosis [31, 32]. The diagnosis of ALS remains fundamentally clinical and relies on the medical history and physical examination. Electrodiagnostic testing with needle electromyography (EMG) and neuroimaging have been useful adjunctive tools in the diagnostic process. EMG provides evidence of LMN involvement, also at subclinical stages, revealing signs of acute denervation like fibrillation potentials, positive sharp waves, and fasciculations. Unfortunately, in cases of UMN-predominant ALS, particularly those with bulbar onset, its sensitivity is still unsatisfactory [33]. Brain and spinal cord magnetic resonance imaging is recommended in order to exclude structural lesions like infarct, cervical radiculomyelopathy, syrinx, demyelination, or neoplasm [34, 35]. Moreover, 18F-fluorodeoxyglucose positron emission tomography (18F-FDG) may reveal a typical pattern of perirolandic and prefrontal hypometabolism [36, 37]. Furthermore, several serum and cerebrospinal fluid molecules, such as neurofilament light chain (NfL) and phosphorylated neurofilament heavy chain (pNfH), are emerging as potential diagnostic and prognostic ALS biomarkers [38].

Genetics plays an important role in the pathophysiology of ALS; in fact, more than forty genes contributing to familial (fALS) and sporadic ALS (sALS) have been identified up to date [39]. The familial form of ALS constitutes up to 10% of disease cases. Familial ALS is most frequently caused by mutations in *C9orf72*, superoxide dismutase 1 gene (*SOD1*), fused of the sarcoma (*FUS*), and *TARDBP* gene [40]. The pattern of inheritance depends on the gene involved and in most cases is autosomal dominant. Mutations in the same genes are also found in sALS patients, but at considerably lower frequencies [41]. The studies of ALS at the molecular level have indicated cytoplasmic aggregation of TAR DNA-binding protein 43 (TDP-43), a protein encoded by *TARDBP*, as the most common ALS neuropathology, present in more than 95% of cases [42]. Except for accumulation of misfolded or aggregated proteins, other cellular processes like oxidative stress, excitotoxicity, mitochondrial dysfunction, endoplasmic reticulum stress, and inflammation can result in the loss of neurons in ALS [43]. Similar abnormalities at the genetic and molecular level have been described in patients with frontotemporal dementia (FTD) [44]. In fact, around 15% of ALS patients meet the criteria of frontotemporal dementia (FTD), and conversely, up to 15% of FTD patients develop ALS [45, 46]. In fact, ALS and FTD may be considered one disease, with ALS representing predominantly motor phenotype and FTD cognitive phenotype [47].

Significant discoveries in genetics research has brought a better understanding of ALS pathogenesis over recent years, which is crucial for the development of disease-modifying and curative therapies in the future [48]. At this point, riluzole remains the only widely approved drug for the treatment of ALS. Riluzole exerts inhibitory effects on the glutamatergic system, which prevents neuronal dysfunction and death called "excitotoxicity." Unfortunately, the benefit is very limited, and riluzole can extend the average survival time by only 3 months [49]. Another drug, edaravone, is a free radical scavenger that reduces oxidative stress. The first clinical trials conducted in Japan and in the USA have shown that the treatment with edaravone may prolong survival up to 6 months, leading to the approval of the drug by several countries [50, 51]. Unfortunately, its beneficial clinical effects have not been confirmed in European cohorts [52, 53]. The third available drug, AMX0035, is a combination of two compounds—tauroursodeoxycholic acid (TUDCA) and sodium phenylbutyrate (PB)—and is believed to increase the threshold for cell death by blocking key cell death pathways. After promising results of the first randomized, placebo-controlled, phase 2 trial of AMX0035 in ALS (CENTAUR), in which the treatment with AMX0035 led to both functional and survival benefits in ALS patients, the drug has been approved in the USA and Canada [54]. The collaborative research efforts do not stop, and there are many experimental therapies in development, targeting, among others, excitotoxicity, oxidative stress, mitochondrial dysfunction, protein homeostasis, and neuroinflammation [55]. Furthermore, cannabis-based medicine has been gaining increasing attention as a potential therapeutic agent for many neurological conditions, including ALS [56–58].

4. Upper motor neuron (UMN) syndromes

Pure upper motor neuron (UMN) syndromes comprise PLS, which as a phenotype of ALS was mentioned above, and hereditary spastic paraplegia (HSP). PLS clinically overlaps with (UMN)-predominant ALS and HSP, posing a diagnostic challenge to the clinicians. Nevertheless, HSP compared to PLS is more frequently associated with the presence of a family history, the earlier and symmetric onset of the disease, diminished vibratory sensation, the absence of bulbar involvement, and slower disease progression [59].

4.1 Hereditary spastic paraplegia (HSP)

Hereditary spastic paraplegia (HSP) describes a heterogeneous group of neurodegenerative diseases with a complex genetic background of more than 70 genetic variants recognized, with all possible patterns of inheritance reported [39]. Between 13 and 40% of cases occur, however, with no family history [60]. Clinically, the "pure" form of HSP is marked by progressive spasticity of the lower limbs, whereas "complex" variants of HSP encompass additional disturbances, including dementia, cognitive delay, epilepsy, neuropathy, and others. The disease can present in infancy, childhood, adolescence, or adulthood. Nonetheless, the more common autosomal-dominant types manifest between the second and third decades [61].

Autosomal dominant hereditary spastic paraplegia 4 (SPG4) is the most prevalent form of HSP. Among the autosomal-recessive forms, SPG11 is the most frequent and associated with a "complex" phenotype [62]. Disease progression in HSP individuals is overall slow. Late disease onset and SPG11 form are associated with a higher disease severity and earlier loss of independent walking. The diagnosis of HSP is made based on clinical features, genetic testing, and neuroimaging. Despite the wide attainability of the next-generation sequencing-based HSP gene panels, a genetic diagnosis is not made in up to 71% of all suspected cases of HSP [60].

Up to this date, no specific HSP modifying therapy is available [63]. Oral antispasmodics, including baclofen and tizanidine, have an established role in the management of spasticity; another promising oral treatment option is fampridine (4-aminopyridine) [64]. In more severe cases, the administration of intrathecal baclofen may be used to alleviate spasticity and improve gait [65]. Sadly, despite great progress in unraveling the genetics of HSP, no substantial advances in developing gene-specific therapy have been achieved [39].

5. Conclusions

Over the last decades, considerable efforts have been made to unfold the underlying pathophysiology of MNDs and find novel therapeutic modalities. Yet MNDs present a unique challenge to researchers and clinicians. The approval of three efficacious and safe therapies (nusinersen, risdiplam, and onasemnogene abeparvovec) led to a breakthrough in the management of SMA. With regard to ALS, diagnostic and prognostic procedures have remained relatively unchanged, apart from genetic testing. Neurofilament light chain and phosphorylated neurofilament heavy chain have emerged as possible diagnostic and prognostic biomarkers in serum and cerebrospinal fluid of the ALS patients. On the other hand, as NfL and pNfH levels are elevated in many neurodegenerative diseases, their clinical utility might be insufficient. Available treatment options for ALS are limited and not curative. Three disease modifying drugs have been approved by the US Food and Drug Administration (FDA), including riluzole, edaravone, and AMX0035. Due to contradictory results in clinical trials, edaravone and AMX0035 have not been approved in most of the European countries. Currently, the multidisciplinary supportive care provided by medical practitioners in neurology, pulmonology, gastroenterology, rehabilitation, and palliative care continues to be the core stone of MND management. Our book aims to discuss the latest developments in the field of MNDs.

Author details

Kamila Saramak[1] and Natalia Szejko[2,3]*

1 Department of Neurology, Hochzirl Hospital, Zirl, Austria

2 Department of Clinical Neurosciences, University of Calgary, Alberta, Canada

3 Department of Bioethics, Medical University of Warsaw, Poland

*Address all correspondence to: natalia.szejko@gmail.com

References

[1] Foster LA, Salajegheh MK. Motor neuron disease: Pathophysiology, diagnosis, and management. The American Journal of Medicine. 2019;**132**:32-37

[2] Statland JM, Barohn RJ, McVey AL, Katz JS, Dimachkie M. Patterns of weakness, classification of motor neuron disease, and clinical diagnosis of sporadic amyotrophic lateral sclerosis. Neurologic Clinics. 2015;**33**:735-748

[3] Barp A, Sansone VA, Lunetta C. Challenges in diagnosis of motor neuron disease: A case series of ALS mimic syndromes. Revue Neurologique. 2021;**177**:699-706

[4] de Carvalho M, Swash M. Diagnosis and differential diagnosis of MND/ ALS: IFCN Handbook Chapter. In: Clinical Neurophysiology Practice. The Netherlands, Amsterdam: Elsevier; 2024;**9**:27-38

[5] Kim W-K, Liu X, Sandner J, Pasmantier M, Andrews J, Rowland L, et al. Study of 962 patients indicates progressive muscular atrophy is a form of ALS. Neurology. 2009;**73**:1686-1692

[6] Mercuri E, Sumner CJ, Muntoni F, Darras BT, Finkel RS. Spinal muscular atrophy. Nature Reviews Disease Primers. 2022;**8**:52

[7] Wirth B, Karakaya M, Kye MJ, Mendoza-Ferreira N. Twenty-five years of spinal muscular atrophy research: From phenotype to genotype to therapy, and what comes next. Annual Review of Genomics and Human Genetics. 2020;**21**:231-261

[8] Mercuri E, Darras BT, Chiriboga CA, Day JW, Campbell C, Connolly AM, et al. Nusinersen versus sham control in later-onset spinal muscular atrophy. New England Journal of Medicine. 2018;**378**:625-635

[9] Finkel RS, Mercuri E, Darras BT, Connolly AM, Kuntz NL, Kirschner J, et al. Nusinersen versus sham control in infantile-onset spinal muscular atrophy. New England Journal of Medicine. 2017;**377**:1723-1732

[10] Day JW, Finkel RS, Chiriboga CA, Connolly AM, Crawford TO, Darras BT, et al. Onasemnogene abeparvovec gene therapy for symptomatic infantile-onset spinal muscular atrophy in patients with two copies of SMN2 (STR1VE): An open-label, single-arm, multicentre, phase 3 trial. The Lancet Neurology. 2021;**20**:284-293

[11] Baranello G, Darras BT, Day JW, Deconinck N, Klein A, Masson R, et al. Risdiplam in type 1 spinal muscular atrophy. New England Journal of Medicine. 2021;**384**:915-923

[12] Darras BT, Masson R, Mazurkiewicz-Bełdzińska M, Rose K, Xiong H, Zanoteli E, et al. Risdiplam-treated infants with type 1 spinal muscular atrophy versus historical controls. New England Journal of Medicine. 2021;**385**:427-435

[13] Antonaci L, Pera MC, Mercuri E. New therapies for spinal muscular atrophy: Where we stand and what is next. European Journal of Pediatrics. 2023;**182**:2935-2942

[14] Oechsel KF, Cartwright MS. Combination therapy with onasemnogene and risdiplam in spinal muscular atrophy type 1. Muscle & Nerve. 2021;**64**:487-490

[15] Shaw SW, Peng S-Y, Liang C-C, Lin T-Y, Cheng P-J, Hsieh T-T, et al. Prenatal transplantation of human amniotic fluid stem cell could improve clinical outcome of type III spinal muscular atrophy in mice. Scientific Reports. 2021;**11**:9158

[16] Han F, Ebrahimi-Barough S, Abolghasemi R, Ai J, Liu Y. Cell-based therapy for spinal muscular atrophy. In: Stem Cell-based Therapy for Neurodegenerative Diseases. Singapore: Springer; 2020;**1266**:117-125

[17] Rhodes LE, Freeman BK, Auh S, Kokkinis AD, La Pean A, Chen C, et al. Clinical features of spinal and bulbar muscular atrophy. Brain. 2009;**132**:3242-3251

[18] Sperfeld AD, Karitzky J, Brummer D, Schreiber H, Häussler J, Ludolph AC, et al. X-linked bulbospinal neuronopathy: Kennedy disease. Archives of Neurology. 2002;**59**:1921-1926

[19] Badders NM, Korff A, Miranda HC, Vuppala PK, Smith RB, Winborn BJ, et al. Selective modulation of the androgen receptor AF2 domain rescues degeneration in spinal bulbar muscular atrophy. Nature Medicine. 2018;**24**:427-437

[20] Mehta P, Raymond J, Punjani R, Han M, Larson T, Kaye W, et al. Prevalence of amyotrophic lateral sclerosis in the United States using established and novel methodologies. Amyotrophic Lateral Sclerosis and Frontotemporal Degeneration. 2017;**2022**:1-9

[21] Park J, Kim J-E, Song T-J. The global burden of motor neuron disease: An analysis of the 2019 global burden of disease study. Frontiers in Neurology. 2022;**13**:864339

[22] Xu L, Liu T, Liu L, Yao X, Chen L, Fan D, et al. Global variation in prevalence and incidence of amyotrophic lateral sclerosis: A systematic review and meta-analysis. Journal of Neurology. 2020;**267**:944-953

[23] Marin B, Boumédiene F, Logroscino G, Couratier P, Babron M-C, Leutenegger AL, et al. Variation in worldwide incidence of amyotrophic lateral sclerosis: A meta-analysis. International journal of epidemiology. 2017;**46**:57-74

[24] Arthur KC, Calvo A, Price TR, Geiger JT, Chio A, Traynor BJ. Projected increase in amyotrophic lateral sclerosis from 2015 to 2040. Nature Communications. 2016;**7**:12408

[25] Turner MR, Barnwell J, Al-Chalabi A, Eisen A. Young-onset amyotrophic lateral sclerosis: Historical and other observations. Brain. 2012;**135**:2883-2891

[26] Chiò A, Calvo A, Moglia C, Mazzini L, Mora G. Phenotypic heterogeneity of amyotrophic lateral sclerosis: A population based study. Journal of Neurology, Neurosurgery & Psychiatry. 2011;**82**:740-746

[27] Fujimura-Kiyono C, Kimura F, Ishida S, Nakajima H, Hosokawa T, Sugino M, et al. Onset and spreading patterns of lower motor neuron involvements predict survival in sporadic amyotrophic lateral sclerosis. Journal of Neurology, Neurosurgery & Psychiatry. 2011;**82**:1244-1249

[28] Stegmann GM, Hahn S, Liss J, Shefner J, Rutkove S, Shelton K, et al. Early detection and tracking of bulbar changes in ALS via frequent and remote speech analysis. NPJ Digital Medicine. 2020;**3**:132

[29] Westeneng H-J, Debray TP, Visser AE, van Eijk RP, Rooney JP,

Calvo A, et al. Prognosis for patients with amyotrophic lateral sclerosis: Development and validation of a personalised prediction model. The Lancet Neurology. 2018;**17**:423-433

[30] Ludolph A, Drory V, Hardiman O, Nakano I, Ravits J, Robberecht W, et al. A revision of the El Escorial criteria-2015. Amyotrophic Lateral Sclerosis & Frontotemporal Degeneration. 2015;**16**:291-292

[31] Turner MR. Diagnosing ALS: The Gold Coast criteria and the role of EMG. Practical Neurology. 2022;**22**:176-178

[32] Pugdahl K, Camdessanché J-P, Cengiz B, de Carvalho M, Liguori R, Rossatto C, et al. Gold Coast diagnostic criteria increase sensitivity in amyotrophic lateral sclerosis. Clinical Neurophysiology. 2021;**132**:3183-3189

[33] Colombo E, Doretti A, Scheveger F, Maranzano A, Pata G, Gagliardi D, et al. Correlation between clinical phenotype and electromyographic parameters in amyotrophic lateral sclerosis. Journal of Neurology. 2023;**270**:511-518

[34] Storti B, Diamanti S, Tremolizzo L, Riva N, Lunetta C, Filippi M, et al. ALS mimics due to affection of the cervical spine: From common compressive myelopathy to rare CSF epidural collection. Case Reports in Neurology. 2021;**13**:145-156

[35] Kassubek J, Pagani M. Imaging in amyotrophic lateral sclerosis: MRI and PET. Current Opinion in Neurology. 2019;**32**:740-746

[36] Pagani M, Chiò A, Valentini MC, Öberg J, Nobili F, Calvo A, et al. Functional pattern of brain FDG-PET in amyotrophic lateral sclerosis. Neurology. 2014;**83**:1067-1074

[37] Van Laere K, Vanhee A, Verschueren J, De Coster L, Driesen A, Dupont P, et al. Value of 18fluorodeoxyglucose–positron-emission tomography in amyotrophic lateral sclerosis: A prospective study. JAMA Neurology. 2014;**71**:553-561

[38] Steinacker P, Feneberg E, Weishaupt J, Brettschneider J, Tumani H, Andersen PM, et al. Neurofilaments in the diagnosis of motoneuron diseases: A prospective study on 455 patients. Journal of Neurology, Neurosurgery & Psychiatry. 2016;**87**:12-20

[39] Shribman S, Reid E, Crosby AH, Houlden H, Warner TT. Hereditary spastic paraplegia: From diagnosis to emerging therapeutic approaches. The Lancet Neurology. 2019;**18**:1136-1146

[40] Mejzini R, Flynn LL, Pitout IL, Fletcher S, Wilton SD, Akkari PA. ALS genetics, mechanisms, and therapeutics: Where are we now? Frontiers in Neuroscience. 2019;**13**:497022

[41] Van Daele SH, Moisse M, van Vugt JJ, Zwamborn RA, van der Spek R, van Rheenen W, et al. Genetic variability in sporadic amyotrophic lateral sclerosis. Brain. 2023;**146**:3760-3769

[42] Neumann M, Sampathu DM, Kwong LK, Truax AC, Micsenyi MC, Chou TT, et al. Ubiquitinated TDP-43 in frontotemporal lobar degeneration and amyotrophic lateral sclerosis. Science. 2006;**314**:130-133

[43] Goutman SA, Hardiman O, Al-Chalabi A, Chió A, Savelieff MG, Kiernan MC, et al. Emerging insights into the complex genetics and pathophysiology of amyotrophic lateral sclerosis. The Lancet Neurology. 2022;**21**:465-479

[44] Burrell JR, Halliday GM, Kril JJ, Ittner LM, Götz J, Kiernan MC, et al.

The frontotemporal dementia-motor neuron disease continuum. The Lancet. 2016;**388**:919-931

[45] Ringholz G, Appel SH, Bradshaw M, Cooke N, Mosnik D, Schulz P. Prevalence and patterns of cognitive impairment in sporadic ALS. Neurology. 2005;**65**:586-590

[46] Phukan J, Elamin M, Bede P, Jordan N, Gallagher L, Byrne S, et al. The syndrome of cognitive impairment in amyotrophic lateral sclerosis: A population-based study. Journal of Neurology, Neurosurgery & Psychiatry. 2012;**83**:102-108

[47] de Carvalho M. Advances in amyotrophic lateral sclerosis research in 2022. The Lancet Neurology. 2023;22:21-2

[48] Chia R, Chiò A, Traynor B. Novel genes associated with amyotrophic lateral sclerosis: Diagnostic and clinical implications. The Lancet Neurology. 2018;**17**:94-102

[49] Bensimon G, Lacomblez L, Meininger V, Group ARS. A controlled trial of riluzole in amyotrophic lateral sclerosis. New England Journal of Medicine. 1994;**330**:585-591

[50] Lacomblez L, Bensimon G, Leigh PN, Guillet P, Meininger V. Dose-ranging study of riluzole in amyotrophic lateral sclerosis. Amyotrophic lateral sclerosis/Riluzole Study Group II. Lancet. 1996;**347**:1425-1431

[51] Abe K, Aoki M, Tsuji S, Itoyama Y, Sobue G, Togo M, et al. Safety and efficacy of edaravone in well defined patients with amyotrophic lateral sclerosis: A randomised, double-blind, placebo-controlled trial. The Lancet Neurology. 2017;**16**:505-512

[52] Witzel S, Maier A, Steinbach R, Grosskreutz J, Koch JC, Sarikidi A, et al. Safety and effectiveness of long-term intravenous administration of edaravone for treatment of patients with amyotrophic lateral sclerosis. JAMA Neurology. 2022;**79**:121-130

[53] Lunetta C, Moglia C, Lizio A, Caponnetto C, Dubbioso R, Giannini F, et al. The Italian multicenter experience with edaravone in amyotrophic lateral sclerosis. Journal of Neurology. 2020;**267**:3258-3267

[54] Paganoni S, Hendrix S, Dickson SP, Knowlton N, Macklin EA, Berry JD, et al. Long-term survival of participants in the CENTAUR trial of sodium phenylbutyrate-taurursodiol in amyotrophic lateral sclerosis. Muscle & Nerve. 2021;**63**:31-39

[55] Jiang J, Wang Y, Deng M. New developments and opportunities in drugs being trialed for amyotrophic lateral sclerosis from 2020 to 2022. Frontiers in Pharmacology;**2022**:13

[56] Saramak K, Szejko N. Endocannabinoid System as a New Therapeutic Avenue for the Treatment of Huntington's Disease. In: From Pathophysiology to Treatment of Huntington's Disease. London, UK: IntechOpen; 2022

[57] Szejko N, Saramak K, Lombroso A, Müller-Vahl K. Cannabis-based medicine in treatment of patients with Gilles de la Tourette syndrome. Neurologia i Neurochirurgia Polska. 2022;**56**:28-38

[58] Saramak K, Szejko N. The Endocannabinoid System as a Potential Therapeutic Target for Amyotrophic Lateral Sclerosis: Motor Neurons – New Insights. London, UK: Intech Open; 2024

[59] Fullam T, Statland J. Upper motor neuron disorders: Primary lateral sclerosis, upper motor neuron dominant

amyotrophic lateral sclerosis, and hereditary spastic paraplegia. Brain Sciences. 2021;**11**:611

[60] Schüle R, Wiethoff S, Martus P, Karle KN, Otto S, Klebe S, et al. Hereditary spastic paraplegia: Clinicogenetic lessons from 608 patients. Annals of Neurology. 2016;**79**:646-658

[61] Harding A. Classification of the hereditary ataxias and paraplegias. The Lancet. 1983;**321**:1151-1155

[62] Varga R-E, Khundadze M, Damme M, Nietzsche S, Hoffmann B, Stauber T, et al. In vivo evidence for lysosome depletion and impaired autophagic clearance in hereditary spastic paraplegia type SPG11. PLoS Genetics. 2015;**11**:e1005454

[63] Bertolucci F, Di Martino S, Orsucci D, Ienco EC, Siciliano G, Rossi B, et al. Robotic gait training improves motor skills and quality of life in hereditary spastic paraplegia. NeuroRehabilitation. 2015;**36**:93-99

[64] Béreau M, Anheim M, Chanson J-B, Tio G, Echaniz-Laguna A, Depienne C, et al. Dalfampridine in hereditary spastic paraplegia: A prospective, open study. Journal of Neurology. 2015;**262**:1285-1288

[65] Margetis K, Korfias S, Boutos N, Gatzonis S, Themistocleous M, Siatouni A, et al. Intrathecal baclofen therapy for the symptomatic treatment of hereditary spastic paraplegia. Clinical Neurology & Neurosurgery. 2014;**123**:142-145

Chapter 2

From Motor Neuron Specification to Function: Filling in the Gaps

Mudassar Nazar Khan and Till Marquardt

Abstract

Motor neurons operate at the interface between nervous system and movement apparatus and play several roles in movement generation. During development, motor neurons emerge from progenitor cells in the ventral neural tube and eventually settle into stereotypic position that predict the identity of their target muscles. The specification of these 'positional' identities has been studied in detail and involves a coordinate grid of intersecting extrinsic signals that result in the activation of unique combinations of transcription factors acting as cell-autonomous determinants. Eventually, motor neurons diversify into 'functional' (e.g., fast/intermediate/slow alpha, beta, and gamma) subtypes essential for proper movement execution, a process linked to the acquisition of unique sets of functional properties. Recent progress has provided insights into the molecular composition and specification of motor neuron functional identities, but little is known about their relationship to the mechanisms underlying the specification of positional identities. In this chapter, we attempt to provide a framework for consolidating both aspects of motor neuron diversification, in addition to outlining the gaps in our knowledge to guide future research directions aiming at understanding the events on a motor neuron's journey from specification to function.

Keywords: spinal motor neurons, motor neuron functional specification, motor neuron positional identities, motor neuron development, neurogenesis, movement control, neuronal development, gamma, beta, alpha motor neurons, fast, slow motor neurons

1. Introduction

To paraphrase Sherrington, motor neurons represent the final common pathway in the generation of behaviors by linking the nervous system with the movement apparatus [1]. This role is reflected by two levels of organization, one spatial and one functional, that together allow motor neurons to serve as the interface through which the brain can engage with and act upon the external world. On the one hand, motor neurons are somatotopically organized, with the position of motor neuron somas in the spinal cord predicting the specific muscle it controls (**Figure 1**) [2]. These 'positional' identities of motor neurons are specified early in development, prior to the establishment of neuromuscular connections [2]. On the other hand, motor neuron diversity is defined by different roles in movement generation and by the different

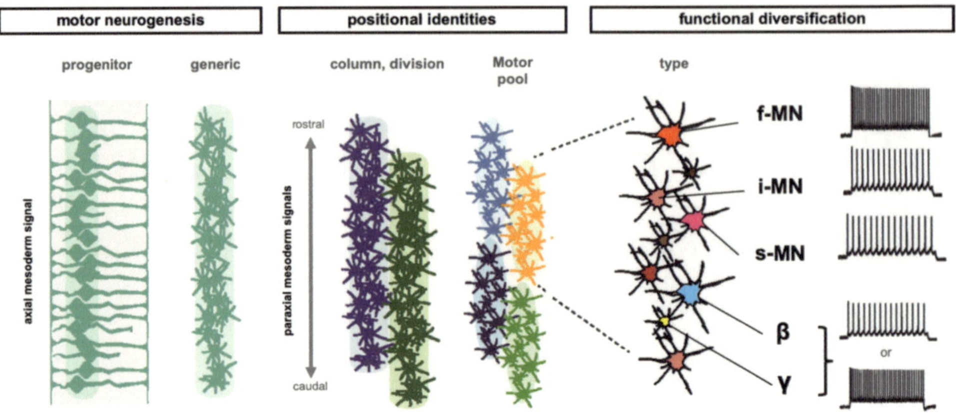

Figure 1.
Schematic summarizing the different levels of motor neuron specification. All spinal motor neurons originate from neuron progenitor cells in the ventral neural tube. Motor neuron positional identities (columns, divisions innervating certain muscle groups and motor pools innervating individual muscles) are acquired after cell-cycle exit. A typical motor pool of tetrapod vertebrates contains a mixture of different 'functional' motor neuron types: Alpha motor neurons (fast/f-MNs, intermediate/i-MNs and slow/s-MNs) as well as beta and gamma motor neurons, which all possess different biophysical properties such as firing rates (such as high firing rates for f-MNs and gamma motor neurons) and roles in movement execution and control. It remains unclear, when exactly motor neuron functional diversity is generated and to what extent, if at all, this is coordinated with the specification of motor pool identities.

muscle fiber types that are innervated (**Figure 1**) [3]. In tetrapod vertebrates, a skeletal muscle typically contains a mixture of different muscle fiber types and is supplied by a range of motor neuron types involved in different aspects of movement generation or control [2, 4–6]. To avoid confusion, we will refer to the first instance of motor neuron diversity as 'positional' diversity and the second as 'functional' diversity. While the mechanisms promoting positional or functional diversity may operate independently form each other, an individual motor neuron can eventually be assigned both by a positional and a functional identity (**Figure 1**). Several excellent reviews have appeared in recent years covering either positional or functional motor neuron diversification [2, 3, 7]. To avoid redundancy, we will in this chapter just briefly touch upon the fundamentals of both spatial and functional motor neuron diversity and mostly focus on what is known—or rather what is not—about the link between the mechanisms that underlie the development of both types of motor neuron diversity necessary for proper movement execution and control.

2. Motor neuron positional identities

2.1 Initial specification of motor neuron identity

Positionally distinct classes of motor neurons emerge in the developing spinal cord whose fates are specified under the influence of intersecting gradients of signaling molecules called morphogens along the dorsoventral (d-v) and rostrocaudal (r-c) axes of the neural tube [8, 9]. Morphogens are secreted from several embryonic structures to the neural tube: Sonic hedgehog (Shh) from the notochord and floor plate and bone morphogenetic protein (BMP) and wingless (Wnt) from the dorsal roof plate and surface ectoderm, retinoic acid (RA) from the paraxial mesoderm and fibroblast growth factors (FGFs) from the caudal mesoderm and tail bud, that together contribute to the specification of molecular identities of neural progenitor cells or domains along the d-v and r-c axes of the neural tube [8, 9]. Shh drives the specification of motor neuron progenitor (pMN) and interneuron populations (V0, V1, V2, V3) in the ventral spinal cord, while RA and FGFs also contribute to motor neuron progenitor identities [10–12]. The graded expression of Shh in the d-v axis regulates Gli (Glioma-associated oncogene) family transcription factors activity, which establishes the neural progenitor domains via the expression of Class I and II homeodomain transcription factors (TFs) [9].

Progenitor domain boundaries develop and are sustained through the cross-repressive actions of class I (Pax7, Pax6, Irx3, Dbx1, Dbx2) and Class II TFs (Nkx6.1 and Nkx2.2) [13]. The co-expression of Pax6 and Nkx6.1 activates the expression of basic helix-basic-helix (bHLH) protein Olig2, which together mark the motor neuron progenitor domain [14–16]. The expression of Olig2 and its repressive activities (specifically, the repression of a repressor that normally represses Ngn2 expression) leads to the indirect upregulation of Ngn2. This results in the expression of post-mitotic motor neuron genes of Lhx3/Isl1 and motor-neuron specific gene Mnx1 (Hb9) [13, 17, 18]. Moreover, the expression levels of Olig2/Ngn2 must be balanced to ensure timely motor neuron specific gene expression, since high expression of Olig2 sustains the pMN state, while high levels of Ngn2 activates the conversion of pMN to post-mitotic motor neurons [19]. Post-mitotic neuron classes, like the progenitor classes, are specified by the combinatorial expression of transcription factors, and in addition, develop specific patterns of connectivity, a neurotransmitter system and electrophysiological properties [8, 9]. Newly born post-mitotic motor neurons express a set of TFs like Lhx3, Isl1 and Mnx1 and send axons peripherally to muscles, use acetylcholine and glutamate as neurotransmitters [20, 21]. This set of early post-mitotic TFs bind to specific enhancers to specify and maintain motor neuron identity [22, 23].

2.2 Specification of motor neuron positional identities: columns, divisions and pools

A second level of motor neuron organization within the spinal cord is the clustering of somas into columns within the r-c axis (**Figure 1**). These positional identities are patterned by reciprocally graded concentrations of fibroblast growth factors (FGFs) and retinoic acid (RA) that regulate the temporal and spatial expression of homeobox (*Hox*) family transcription factors [24–26]. *Hox* family transcription factors are sequentially arranged on chromosomes in four clusters (*HoxA, HoxB, HoxC, HoxD*) that encode 39 genes that are expressed in the spinal cord and hindbrain during both progenitor and post-mitotic phases of motor neuron differentiation [27, 28]. RA regulates the expression of *Hox4-Hox6* genes at the cervical/brachial levels of the spinal cord [7, 26]. While FGF induces *Hox4-Hox10* in cervical/brachial, thoracic and lumbar levels of the spinal cord and Gdf11/FGF8 induce *Hox10* in the lumbar spinal cord [7, 26].

Hox gene expression pattern in post-mitotic motor neurons determines their columnar subtype identity. For example, in the phrenic motor column (PMC), motor neurons at the cervical level of the spinal cord express *Hox5* [29]. Loss of *Hox5* in motor neurons results in failure of dendritic arborization in the diaphragm muscle and neuronal death leading to respiratory failure and perinatal death in mice [29]. The lumbar motor column (LMC) motor neurons of the brachial and lumbar levels express *Hox6* and *Hox10*, respectively [25, 30–34]. The specification of LMC depends on the expression of *Hox* genes and their regulation of Foxp1 expression pattern [30, 32]. The preganglionic motor column (PGC) motor neuron identities depend on *Hoxc9* expression [35]. While, motor neurons that innervate axial muscles do not depend on *Hox* gene programs. For example, the medial motor column (MMC) columnar subtype motor neurons identity depends on the *Wnt* genes and are marked by the expression of Prdm family transcription factor Mecom [7, 36, 37]. Still, the programs involved in the specification of other motor columns, like hypaxial motor column (HMC) which innervates axial muscles are unknown.

A third level of motor neuron organization is known as divisional identity which is defined by the motor axons and the muscles they target. The genetic programs that are involved in the specification of muscle targets have been studied extensively in the lateral motor column (LMC) motor neurons. While the generation of LMC motor neurons depends on *Hox* genes and the expression pattern of transcription factors they regulate, the maturation of LMC neurons is dependent on both the limb-derived cues and molecular programs intrinsic to motor neurons. *Hox* genes promote high *Foxp1* expression levels, which is required for the expression of Raldh2, an enzyme that catalyzes retinoic acid (RA) synthesis. Localized synthesis of RA in motor neurons at the brachial and lumbar spinal cord levels establish LMC divisional identities [38–40]. The LMC motor neurons express specific Lim homeodomain (HD) proteins and their axons target specific muscles groups of the limbs, which confers their divisional identity: the lateral division (LMCl) motor neurons express Lhx1 and send axons to the muscles within the dorsal compartment, while the medial division (LMCm) motor neurons express Isl1 and send axons to the muscles within the dorsal compartment [41]. To ensure LMCl identity, Lhx1 expression is maintained by the repressive interaction between Lhx1 and Isl1, the protein signaling controlled by the sources of RA from Raldh2$^+$ motor neuron and the paraxial mesoderm [7, 38–40]. Moreover, the routes that LMCl motor neuron axons select within the limbs is dependent upon Lhx1 expression. Lhx1 expression within LMCl regulates the expression of axonal guidance receptor Eph4 (which repels ventral axons that express ephrin), leading to the dorsal projection of axons [7, 42, 43]. Moreover, ventrally projecting LMCm axons use similar signaling strategies: Lim HD proteins regulate the expression of axonal guidance molecules like ephrin and Eph receptors that ultimately determine axonal trajectories [7, 44].

A fourth level of motor neuron organization observed in the spinal cord are motor pools (**Figure 1**). Motor neurons within a specific motor pool cluster in a specific position in the spinal cord, innervate a single muscle, have specific type (alpha/gamma) ratios and show motor pool-specific molecular marker expression, morphology, central and peripheral connectivity, and electrophysiological patterns. These features are determined by *Hox* genes, in part, and by molecular cues from peripheral targets. Early on in development, motor pool diversity is regulated by *Hox* genes and their regulation of transcription factor expression levels. Combinatorial expression of *Hoxc8* and *Hoxc6* determines the expression of several proteins, including ETS domain transcription factor Pea3, the Pou domain protein Scip (also known as Pou3f1), and Nkx6.1, which ultimately characterize LMC motor pool identities [7]. Thus, the loss of *Hoxc8* and *Hoxc6* in mice leads to the decrease in Pea3-expressing motor neurons and decrease in axonal arborization of targeted muscles [31, 45, 46]. Moreover, specific muscle innervation in mice is disrupted in motor pools that no longer express Nkx6.1, a downstream target of *Hox* signaling [47], while *Foxp1* mutant mice show reduced expression of motor pool markers *Pea3*, *Scip* and *Nkx6.1* [32]. Motor pool identities are also regulated by the molecular cues from peripheral muscles. For example, neurotrophic factors like glial-derived neurotrophic factor (GDNF), regulate the expression of Pea3 and thus, determine motor pool soma position and motor pool targeted muscle innervation [48].

3. Motor neuron functional identities

3.1 Motor neuron functional diversity: alpha, beta and gamma motor neurons

The mammalian spinal cord displays a diverse population of motor neurons which is correlated with the heterogeneity of the muscle fiber types they innervate (**Figure 1**). Motor neurons within the mammalian spinal cord can be categorized into functionally diverse classes and subtypes based on several properties: size and morphology, electrical properties, molecular marker expression and function. Based on these characteristics, motor neurons can be divided into three main types, alpha motor neurons (α-MNs), beta motor neurons (β-MNs) and gamma motor neurons (γ-MNs) and several subtypes. Somatic α-MNs exclusively innervate extrafusal muscle fibers that regulate muscle force and movement. While gamma motor neurons innervate the smaller intrafusal fibers located within the muscle spindle proprioceptive organs, regulate the sensory information reported during muscle stretch from the muscle spindle, and thereby contribute to motor control. And beta motor neuron, innervate both extrafusal and intrafusal fibers, and may contribute to both muscle contraction and sensory information gathered from muscle spindles during muscle stretch, although their exact functional contribution remains unknown.

3.2 Alpha motor neurons

Motor neurons and the muscle fibers their axons innervate display a spectrum of properties that are used to categorize them into subtypes. For instance, there is exquisite matching of muscle contractile properties such as isometric twitch speed, maximum force and endurance and alpha motor neuron properties like size and morphology, excitability and firing pattern, which together allow them to contract synchronously as a "motor unit" to drive muscle contraction [49, 50]. Alpha motor units can be classified into three subtypes: (1) slow-twitch fatigue resistant (S), fast-twitch fatigue-resistant (FR), and fast-twitch fatigable (FF) [51]. Each of these motor units possesses a spectrum of properties: S-type are made of type I muscle fibers that contract slow, develop small quantity of force and are very fatigue-resistant, FR-type are comprised of type IIA fibers that contract faster, develop more force and are less fatigue-resistant than the S-type, while the FF-type are made of type IIB fibers that contract the fastest, develop the highest force and are highly fatigable [50, 51].

Alpha motor neurons, which comprise of one-third of motor neurons in a given motor pool, can be identified based on their size and morphology, excitability, biophysical properties, and the expression of molecular markers. Alpha motor neurons are sequentially activated depending on two linked properties of their cell membrane, that is their soma size and morphology (dendritic arborization) and intrinsic properties (quantity and diversity of ion channels) [52, 53]. For example, as a motor pool receives information from descending inputs for eliciting the contraction of the muscle it innervates, S-type motor neurons, possessing smaller soma sizes and more simple dendritic arborization, are activated first because: (1) they possess a higher input resistance, meaning a larger change in cell membrane voltage over constant current injection, and

(2) a lower threshold due to cell membrane Na^+ ion channel sensitivity. Thus, S-type motor neurons fire action potentials with lower synaptic current when compared to the larger FF-type motor neurons. Thus, this sequential activation from S-type motor neuron to FF-type motor neuron is thought to follow Henneman's "size principle" and has implications for motor unit recruitment [54, 55]. Moreover, FR-type motor neurons and motor units have intermediate characteristics between S- and FF-subtypes. Thus, activities that require sustained muscle contraction (standing or walking) results in the recruitment of S-type motor neurons that activate slow motor units, while activities that require potent bursts of muscle contraction (running or jumping) initiates FF-type motor neurons recruitment and subsequent activation of fast motor units, elegantly matching motor neuron morphology and electrical properties with motor unit size required for specific movement tasks [56].

Since motor neurons fire repetitive action potentials, their firing rate can be used to classify them. The firing rate is shaped by persistent inward currents (PICs) generated by voltage-gated Na^+ and Ca^{2+} currents, which are prolonged on dendrites of S-type motor neurons than FF-type motor neurons [57]. PICs amplify and limit the modulation of firing rate, making the S-type motor neurons highly excitable with an initial steep firing rate and subsequent saturation [57]. Another property that determines motor neuron firing rate is the after-hyperpolarization (AHP) phase after the action potential, which is generated by Ca^{2+}-dependent K^+ currents. The influx of Ca^{2+} during the firing of action potentials and the intracellular diffusion, pumping and interaction with proteins regulates AHP-decay times [58–60]. Thus, FF-type motor neurons have a shorter AHP-decay time, therefore a higher maximum firing frequency than S-type motor neurons, which ultimately matches the contractile frequency of the muscle fiber type these motor neurons innervate [3, 61, 62].

Alpha motor neuron subtypes can also be distinguished by the expression of a subset of genes. For instance, studies have shown that FF-type motor neurons express: Calcitonin gene-related peptide (CGRP)/calca, Chondrolectin, Matrix metallopeptidase 9 (MMP-9), and Delta-like homolog 1 (Dlk1) [63–67]. While a synaptic vesicle protein, SV2a is expressed postnatally in presynaptic terminals of S-type motor neurons that innervate type I and small type IIA muscle fibers [68]. Moreover, a study in rat showed that Ca^{2+}-activated K^+ (SK) channels are expressed in S-type alpha motor neurons and the electrophysiological recordings of these $SK3^+$ motor neurons showed medium size AHP-duration, which seems to be in the range of S-type alpha motor neurons [69]. Other putative markers that are expressed in all three alpha motor neuron subtypes (FF, FR and S) are Hb9::GFP, NeuN, Osteopontin, and Na^+/K^+ ATPase (Atp1a1 and Atp1a3) (both alpha 1 and 3 isoforms in FF- and FR-subtypes), while UCHL1::eGFP and Na^+/K^+ ATPase (alpha 1 isoform only) are expressed in S-type [70–77].

3.3 Beta motor neurons

Another class of motor neuron, the beta motor neurons, were thought to exist only in lower vertebrates such as reptiles, amphibians and birds but are also shown to exist in mammals and comprise one-third of all motor units and innervate three-fourths of all muscle spindles [3, 78, 79]. Despite their abundance in quantity, limited anatomical and functional characterization suggests that beta motor neurons possess intermediate properties between alpha and gamma motor neurons and may play important roles in regulating motor behavior. Unlike alpha and gamma motor neurons which exclusively innervate extrafusal and intrafusal fibers, respectively, beta motor neurons innervate both extrafusal and intrafusal fibers, and thus, regulate both muscle contraction and sensory information from the muscle spindle [78]. Based on their hybrid innervation pattern, beta motor neurons can be subdivided into two subtypes: static and dynamic. Static beta motor neurons innervate type IIa extrafusal fibers and bag2 intrafusal fibers, while dynamic motor neurons innervate type I extrafusal fibers and bag1 intrafusal fibers [3]. Thus, the functional role of beta motor neurons is currently unresolved, however, based on their anatomical properties, they seem to play a role in movement and maintenance of posture [3]. Moreover, studies that aim to identify molecular marker expression and electrophysiological properties of beta motor neurons are especially needed in testing what type of functional role they may play in movement and movement control.

3.4 Gamma motor neurons

Like the alpha motor neurons, gamma motor neuron subtypes can be classified based on their distinct patterns of morphology, connectivity, electrical and functional properties. In mammals, gamma motor neurons represent about one-third of the motor neurons in a given spinal motor pool and are distinguished by their singular role of regulating muscle spindle sensitivity and motor control. Gamma motor rely on GDNF secreted from muscle spindle sensory receptors buried deep within skeletal muscle for their postnatal survival, although it is not known how they survive before maturation [70]. Gamma motor neurons innervate the intrafusal fibers within the muscle spindle and receive presynaptic input from sensory neurons within the muscle spindles. Thus, gamma motor neurons enable continuous flow of sensory information about muscle length and ensure fluid muscular action during muscular contractions [6, 80]. Gamma motor neurons can be subdivided into two types based on their intrafusal fiber innervation patterns and their role in regulating muscle spindle sensory information. Dynamic gamma motor neurons innervate bag1 intrafusal fibers and are thought to regulate muscle length during locomotion, while static gamma motor neurons innervate bag2 and nuclear chain fibers and are thought to be involved in body posture [81].

Gamma motor neurons possess unique biophysical properties which were identified based on intracellular and patch clamp recordings in different animal models. Early on, intracellular recordings in the ventral spinal cord of the cat identified that gamma motor neurons had slower conduction velocity (since they have small axon diameter) compared to alpha motor neurons [82–84]. Moreover, studies showed that gamma motor neurons possess lower discharge threshold, higher discharge rates and lower membrane input resistance when compared to alpha motor neurons [85]. Furthermore, gamma motor neuron subtypes display unique firing properties: dynamic gamma motor neurons increase the discharge rate of primary sensory afferents when muscle is stretched, while static gamma motor neurons seem to have no effect on primary sensory afferent firing [86]. Studies in mice have also characterized gamma motor neuron electrophysiological properties. Immature gamma motor neurons in young mice (P0-P6) expressing GFP under serotonin receptor 1d (5-ht1d) promoter were patch clamped and revealed that gamma motor neuron electrical properties of rheobase current, input resistance and AHP-decay time ranged between FF-type and S-type alpha motor neurons [87]. In a recent study, more mature gamma motor neurons from mice (P20–22) labeled with high levels of Fluorogold (FG) (retrograde tracer) showed low rheobase current, high firing frequencies and gain when compared to alpha motor neurons [88]. This study matches some of the gamma motor neuron signature properties observed in the cat.

3.5 Mechanisms underlying motor neuron functional diversification

Differences in the connectivity and physiological properties of motor neurons were first reported in the 1940s and 1950s [84, 89–91], and the significance of these differences have been recognized soon afterwards [6, 84, 92]. Beta and gamma motor neurons were described a few years later [84, 93, 94], and their discovery together significantly broadened our understanding of the neuromuscular bases of movement control and have become canonical topics of neurobiology and neurophysiology textbooks. It therefore seems astonishing that it took over 60 years until the first mechanisms promoting motor neuron functional diversification were discovered [67, 88, 95, 96]. This is likely explained by the difficulties in discovering molecular markers for functional motor neuron types in tetrapod vertebrates due to their general lack of correlation with fixed anatomical features.

Since the first molecular markers for functional motor neuron types were reported, it then took another couple of years until first insights into the mechanisms promoting the diversification of alpha motor neurons into fast and slow types were reported. Herein, the type I transmembrane protein and non-canonical Notch ligand Delta-like homolog 1 (DLK1) was shown to be both necessary and sufficient to promote fast alpha motor neuron gene expression and biophysical signatures required for peak force execution [67]. DLK1 appears to operate in part through the activation of regulatory ion channel subunits including *Kcng4*/KV6.3/4, apparently reflecting its requirement for both specification as well as maturation of fast alpha motor neurons (**Figure 2**) [67]. The transition between initial specification and maturation of

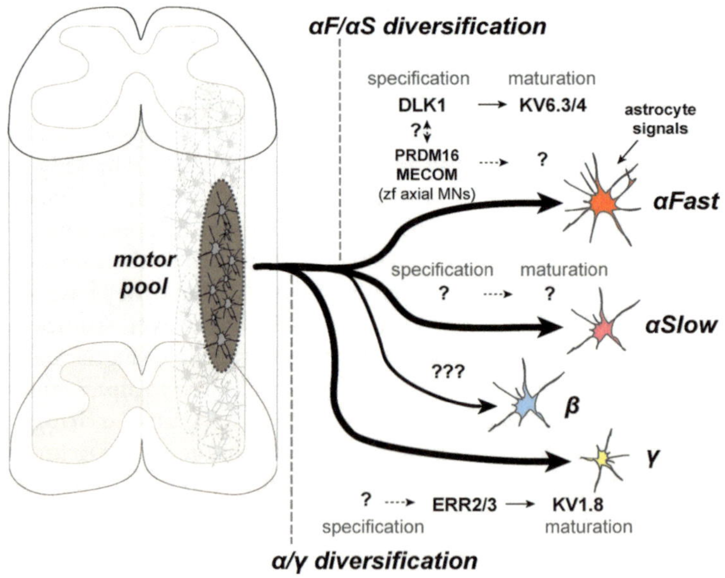

Figure 2.
Schematic summarizing mechanisms identified so far promoting motor neuron functional diversification. While mechanisms promote the acquisition of motor neuron positional identities (not shown) and the organization into different motor pools, parallel or subsequent mechanisms promote the diversification of motor neurons into different alpha, beta and gamma motor neuron types and subtypes. Cell-autonomous mechanisms have been identified underlying the specification and/or maturation alpha and gamma motor neuron types and subtypes, while the maintenance of some alpha motor neuron properties appear to rely on non-cell-autonomous signals by ventral horn astrocytes. Mechanisms underlying the specification of slow alpha motor neurons and beta motor neurons remain to be identified.

motor neurons is further reflected by global shifts in gene expression and chromatin accessibility for different transcription factor classes [97].

More recent work identified two transcription factors PRDM16 and MECOM as early determinants of primary and fast secondary motor neurons in zebrafish, which are likely homologous to tetrapod fast alpha motor neurons [96]. Both transcription factors broadly, but not completely, regulate fast motor neuron gene expression, raising the question of how these molecules are linked to the actions of DLK1 and Notch signaling (**Figure 2**) [96]. The incorporation of neurons into functional circuitries entails not only their specification but also their maturation including the acquisition of specific membrane electrical and firing properties [98]. An intriguing non-cell-autonomous mechanism was found to promote and maintain the mature state of fast alpha motor neuron properties [95]. The potassium channel subunit KIR4.1 expressed by ventral horn astrocytes appears to be required for maintaining fast alpha motor neuron soma size and function through the paracrine activation of mTOR signaling (**Figure 2**) [95]. Again, it remains to be determined how these cell-autonomous (DLK1, PRDM16, MECOM) and non-cell-autonomous mechanisms intersect during alpha motor neuron diversification and maturation (**Figure 2**).

4. Phylogenetic considerations

The spinal motor systems of fish and tetrapod vertebrates differ in key aspects that reflect adaptations specific to swimming and terrestrial locomotion. For instance, fish generally lack muscle spindles and consequently lack gamma or beta motor neurons regulating muscle spindle proprioception [99]. The appearance of muscle spindle and fusimotor systems providing and regulating muscle proprioception obviously represent adaptations to terrestrial locomotion. Another difference between fish and tetrapods is the spatial arrangement of the force-generating alpha motor neurons in the spinal cord. In zebrafish, these neurons are organized into distinct motor columns presynaptically connected to dedicated interneuron modules and postsynaptically to muscle groups containing either slow, intermediate or fast muscle fiber types [100–103]. This arrangement allows rapid transitions from slow undulating swimming to fast escape movements and is apparently adapted to pelagic locomotion. Zebrafish larvae initially possess only fast muscle fibers and primary motor neurons facilitating escape swimming movements, while intermediate and slow muscle fibers and matching secondary motor neuron subtypes are generated later during the transition to adulthood.

The modular architecture of motor neuron subtypes in fish contrasts with that found in tetrapods [102], particularly in mammals, in which most motor pools comprise a mosaic of motor neuron types, including the different alpha motor neuron types, gamma motor neurons and small numbers of beta motor neurons [3]. Exceptions can be found in motor pools connecting to specialized muscles, such as predominantly slow antigravity muscles like the *m. soleus* of the calf or muscles involved in explosive force generation [104], such as the *m. rectus femoris* of the thigh, which are enriched in slow or fast alpha motor neurons, respectively [67]. Moreover, some muscles in birds and non-avian reptiles display regionalized abundances of slow or fast muscle fibers, which are reflected by similar spatial separation of alpha motor neuron types in the corresponding motor pools. Moreover, particularly in primates, motor pools supplying distal forelimb muscles involved in dexterous movements tend to be enriched in gamma motor neurons. Nevertheless, in mammals, and tetrapod vertebrates in general, motor neuron types within the motor pools typically intermingle and do not spatially segregate, as do the fiber types in the skeletal muscles.

While a degree of conservation of the mechanisms underlying the specification of alpha motor neuron types and the axial motor neurons of fish are expected, it is likely that the transition to mosaic organization of motor pools in tetrapods will be reflected by differences in the mechanisms of specification and functional specializations of alpha motor neuron types. In mouse, for instance, DLK1 promotes a gene expression signature specific for fast alpha motor neurons [67], which, however, shows little overlap with that promoted by PRDM16 and MECOM in zebrafish primary and fast secondary motor neurons [96]. While these discrepancies may in part stem from differences in the transcriptome profiling methodologies used by both studies, it is likely that the spatial and functional reorganization of functional motor neuron types in tetrapods reflects an underlying reorganization of genetic circuitries promoting alpha motor neuron diversification.

A similar difference concerns the molecular profile of slow alpha and gamma motor neurons, with slow secondary motor neurons in zebrafish apparently expressing ERR2. In mouse and chick, high levels of ERR2 (together with its paralogue ERR3) mark gamma motor neurons, while lower levels are initially also expressed by alpha motor neurons [65, 71, 88, 96]. It is therefore tempting to speculate that tetrapod fusimotor (beta and gamma) motor neurons evolved from slow motor neurons with a genetic program that enhanced certain sets of preconfigured properties, such as low firing thresholds and small soma sizes. Intriguingly, while fish trunk muscles lack muscle spindles [99], the jaw muscles of some fishes possess muscle-spindle like structures likely supporting rapid prey capture and manipulation movements [105]. It will be highly interesting to test whether such spindle-like structures would receive innervation from motor neurons and how such hypothetical 'ancestral' beta motor neurons would differ in their gene expression profile from axial motor neurons.

5. Conclusions

The two aspects motor neuron diversity discussed in this chapter raise the question of whether both are coordinated and if yes, how? At first glance, both types of motor neuron identity, positional and functional, appear to be established independently form each other. In tetrapod vertebrates, a typical motor pool contains a complement of alpha, beta and gamma motor neuron types and subtypes. Developing motor neurons eventually coalesce into motor pools under the influence of both cell-intrinsic and axon target-induced mechanisms, which in addition to positioning motor neuron somas shape dendritic arbors and presynaptic connectivity. Thus, subsets of motor neurons must somehow acquire distinct sets of properties overlayed on these motor pool-specific features. Moreover, some motor pools are enriched in certain functional motor neuron types mirroring the enrichment in certain fiber types in the muscle they supply. This suggests at least some degree of coordination or crosstalk between motor neuron and muscle fiber type diversification, which is supported by the mutual influence motor neuron and muscle fiber types have on each other. However, this mutual influence only seems to work to some degree, as the conversion of motor neurons from one type to another does not lead to a complete conversion to the corresponding muscle fiber type and *vice versa*. Moreover, there are several lines of evidence that the initial specification of both motor neuron and muscle fiber types occurs in a cell-autonomous fashion but that they to some degree (yet not completely) remain sculptable throughout later life. This initial cell-autonomy suggests that there may be some intersection between the interpretation of positional signal by motor neurons and the eventual generation of certain ratios of motor neuron types, such as the relative abundance of slow motor neuron and muscle fiber types in the *soleus* motor pool and muscle, respectively. There are therefore many open questions remaining, not only regarding the functional diversification of motor neurons but also regarding to what degree and how the underlying mechanisms are coordinated with those promoting motor neuron positional identities.

Acknowledgements

We thank Louisa-Carole Neumann and Dr. Daniel Müller for help and suggestions.

Author details

Mudassar Nazar Khan[1*] and Till Marquardt[2*]

1 Leibniz-Forschungsinstitut für Molekulare Pharmakologie (FMP), Berlin, Germany

2 Faculty for Mathematics, Informatics and Natural Sciences, Clinic for Neurology, RWTH Aachen University Medical Center (UKA), Institute for Biology 2, Aachen, Germany

*Address all correspondence to: khan@fmp-berlin.de and tmarquardt@ukaachen.de

References

[1] Levine DN. Sherrington's "the integrative action of the nervous system": A centennial appraisal. Journal of the Neurological Sciences. 2007;**253**(1-2):1-6. DOI: 10.1016/j.jns.2006.12.002. Epub 2007 Jan 12

[2] Catela C, Shin MM, Dasen JS. Assembly and function of spinal circuits for motor control. Annual Review of Cell and Developmental Biology. 2015;**31**:669-698. DOI: 10.1146/annurev-cellbio-100814-125155. Epub 2015 Sep 21

[3] Manuel M, Zytnicki D. Alpha, beta and gamma motoneurons: Functional diversity in the motor system's final pathway. Journal of Integrative Neuroscience. 2011;**10**(3):243-276. DOI: 10.1142/S0219635211002786

[4] Barnard EA, Lyles JM, Pizzey JA. Fibre types in chicken skeletal muscles and their changes in muscular dystrophy. The Journal of Physiology. 1982;**331**:333-354. DOI: 10.1113/jphysiol.1982.sp014375

[5] Laidlaw DH, Callister RJ, Stuart DG. Fiber-type composition of hindlimb muscles in the turtle, Pseudemys (Trachemys) scripta elegans. Journal of Morphology. 1995;**225**(2):193-211. DOI: 10.1002/jmor.1052250205

[6] Murthy KS. Vertebrate fusimotor neurones and their influences on motor behavior. Progress in Neurobiology. 1978;**11**(3-4):249-307. DOI: 10.1016/0301-0082(78)90015-1

[7] Dasen JS. Establishing the molecular and functional diversity of spinal motoneurons. Advances in Neurobiology. 2022;**28**:3-44. DOI: 10.1007/978-3-031-07167-6_1

[8] Jessell TM. Neuronal specification in the spinal cord: Inductive signals and transcriptional codes. Nature Reviews. Genetics. 2000;**1**(1):20-29. DOI: 10.1038/35049541

[9] Shirasaki R, Pfaff SL. Transcriptional codes and the control of neuronal identity. Annual Review of Neuroscience. 2002;**25**:251-281. DOI: 10.1146/annurev.neuro.25.112701.142916. Epub 2002 Mar 27

[10] Ericson J, Rashbass P, Schedl A, Brenner-Morton S, Kawakami A, van Heyningen V, et al. Pax6 controls progenitor cell identity and neuronal fate in response to graded Shh signaling. Cell. 1997;**90**(1):169-180. DOI: 10.1016/s0092-8674(00)80323-2

[11] Ericson J, Briscoe J, Rashbass P, van Heyningen V, Jessell TM. Graded sonic hedgehog signaling and the specification of cell fate in the ventral neural tube. Cold Spring Harbor Symposia on Quantitative Biology. 1997;**62**:451-466

[12] Novitch BG, Wichterle H, Jessell TM, Sockanathan S. A requirement for retinoic acid-mediated transcriptional activation in ventral neural patterning and motor neuron specification. Neuron. 2003;**40**(1):81-95. DOI: 10.1016/j.neuron.2003.08.006

[13] Briscoe J, Pierani A, Jessell TM, Ericson J. A homeodomain protein code specifies progenitor cell identity and neuronal fate in the ventral neural tube. Cell. 2000;**101**(4):435-445. DOI: 10.1016/s0092-8674(00)80853-3

[14] Novitch BG, Chen AI, Jessell TM. Coordinate regulation of motor neuron subtype identity and pan-neuronal properties by the bHLH repressor Olig2. Neuron. 2001;**31**(5):773-789. DOI: 10.1016/s0896-6273(01)00407-x

[15] Marquardt T, Pfaff SL. Cracking the transcriptional code for cell specification in the neural tube. Cell. 2001;**106**(6):651-654. DOI: 10.1016/s0092-8674(01)00499-8

[16] Zhou Q, Anderson DJ. The bHLH transcription factors OLIG2 and OLIG1 couple neuronal and glial subtype specification. Cell. 2002;**109**(1):61-73. DOI: 10.1016/s0092-8674(02)00677-3

[17] Lee SK, Pfaff SL. Synchronization of neurogenesis and motor neuron specification by direct coupling of bHLH and homeodomain transcription factors. Neuron. 2003;**38**(5):731-745. DOI: 10.1016/s0896-6273(03)00296-4

[18] Ma YC, Song MR, Park JP, Henry Ho HY, Hu L, Kurtev MV, et al. Regulation of motor neuron specification by phosphorylation of neurogenin 2. Neuron. 2008;**58**(1):65-77. DOI: 10.1016/j.neuron.2008.01.037

[19] Lee SK, Lee B, Ruiz EC, Pfaff SL. Olig2 and Ngn2 function in opposition to modulate gene expression in motor neuron progenitor cells. Genes & Development. 2005;**19**(2):282-294. DOI: 10.1101/gad.1257105

[20] Mentis GZ, Alvarez FJ, Bonnot A, Richards DS, Gonzalez-Forero D, Zerda R, et al. Noncholinergic excitatory actions of motoneurons in the neonatal mammalian spinal cord. Proceedings of the National Academy of Sciences of the United States of America. 2005;**102**(20):7344-7349. DOI: 10.1073/pnas.0502788102. Epub 2005 May 9

[21] Nishimaru H, Restrepo CE, Ryge J, Yanagawa Y, Kiehn O. Mammalian motor neurons corelease glutamate and acetylcholine at central synapses. Proceedings of the National Academy of Sciences of the United States of America. 2005;**102**(14):5245-5249. DOI: 10.1073/pnas.0501331102. Epub 2005 Mar 21

[22] Rhee HS, Closser M, Guo Y, Bashkirova EV, Tan GC, Gifford DK, et al. Expression of terminal effector genes in mammalian neurons is maintained by a dynamic relay of transient enhancers. Neuron. 2016;**92**(6):1252-1265. DOI: 10.1016/j.neuron.2016.11.037. Epub 2016 Dec 8

[23] Velasco S, Ibrahim MM, Kakumanu A, Garipler G, Aydin B, Al-Sayegh MA, et al. A multi-step transcriptional and chromatin state cascade underlies motor neuron programming from embryonic stem cells. Cell Stem Cell. 2017;**20**(2):205-217.e8. DOI: 10.1016/j.stem.2016.11.006. Epub 2016 Dec 8

[24] Bel-Vialar S, Itasaki N, Krumlauf R. Initiating Hox gene expression: In the early chick neural tube differential sensitivity to FGF and RA signaling subdivides the HoxB genes in two distinct groups. Development. 2002;**129**(22):5103-5115. DOI: 10.1242/dev.129.22.5103

[25] Dasen JS, Liu JP, Jessell TM. Motor neuron columnar fate imposed by sequential phases of Hox-c activity. Nature. 2003;**425**(6961):926-933. DOI: 10.1038/nature02051

[26] Liu JP, Laufer E, Jessell TM. Assigning the positional identity of spinal motor neurons: Rostrocaudal patterning of Hox-c expression by FGFs, Gdf11, and retinoids. Neuron. 2001;**32**(6):997-1012. DOI: 10.1016/s0896-6273(01)00544-x

[27] Parker HJ, Krumlauf R. A Hox gene regulatory network for hindbrain segmentation. Current Topics in Developmental Biology. 2020;**139**:169-203. DOI: 10.1016/bs.ctdb.2020.03.001. Epub 2020 Apr 9

[28] Philippidou P, Dasen JS. Hox genes: Choreographers in neural

development, architects of circuit organization. Neuron. 2013;**80**(1):12-34. DOI: 10.1016/j.neuron.2013.09.020. Epub 2013 Oct 2

[29] Philippidou P, Walsh CM, Aubin J, Jeannotte L, Dasen JS. Sustained Hox5 gene activity is required for respiratory motor neuron development. Nature Neuroscience. 2012;**15**(12):1636-1644. DOI: 10.1038/nn.3242. Epub 2012 Oct 28

[30] Dasen JS, De Camilli A, Wang B, Tucker PW, Jessell TM. Hox repertoires for motor neuron diversity and connectivity gated by a single accessory factor, FoxP1. Cell. 2008;**134**(2):304-316. DOI: 10.1016/j.cell.2008.06.019

[31] Lacombe J, Hanley O, Jung H, Philippidou P, Surmeli G, Grinstein J, et al. Genetic and functional modularity of Hox activities in the specification of limb-innervating motor neurons. PLoS Genetics. 2013;**9**(1):e1003184. DOI: 10.1371/journal.pgen.1003184. Epub 2013 Jan 24

[32] Rousso DL, Gaber ZB, Wellik D, Morrisey EE, Novitch BG. Coordinated actions of the forkhead protein Foxp1 and Hox proteins in the columnar organization of spinal motor neurons. Neuron. 2008;**59**(2):226-240. DOI: 10.1016/j.neuron.2008.06.025

[33] Shah V, Drill E, Lance-Jones C. Ectopic expression of Hoxd10 in thoracic spinal segments induces motoneurons with a lumbosacral molecular profile and axon projections to the limb. Developmental Dynamics. 2004;**231**(1):43-56. DOI: 10.1002/dvdy.20103

[34] Wu Y, Wang G, Scott SA, Capecchi MR. Hoxc10 and Hoxd10 regulate mouse columnar, divisional and motor pool identity of lumbar motoneurons. Development. 2008;**135**(1):171-182. DOI: 10.1242/dev.009225

[35] Jung H, Lacombe J, Mazzoni EO, Liem KF Jr, Grinstein J, Mahony S, et al. Global control of motor neuron topography mediated by the repressive actions of a single hox gene. Neuron. 2010;**67**(5):781-796. DOI: 10.1016/j.neuron.2010.08.008

[36] Agalliu D, Takada S, Agalliu I, McMahon AP, Jessell TM. Motor neurons with axial muscle projections specified by Wnt4/5 signaling. Neuron. 2009;**61**(5):708-720. DOI: 10.1016/j.neuron.2008.12.026

[37] Hanley O, Zewdu R, Cohen LJ, Jung H, Lacombe J, Philippidou P, et al. Parallel Pbx-dependent pathways govern the coalescence and fate of motor columns. Neuron. 2016;**91**(5):1005-1020. DOI: 10.1016/j.neuron.2016.07.043. Epub 2016 Aug 25

[38] Ji SJ, Zhuang B, Falco C, Schneider A, Schuster-Gossler K, Gossler A, et al. Mesodermal and neuronal retinoids regulate the induction and maintenance of limb innervating spinal motor neurons. Developmental Biology. 2006;**297**(1):249-261. DOI: 10.1016/j.ydbio.2006.05.015. Epub 2006 May 19

[39] Kania A, Johnson RL, Jessell TM. Coordinate roles for LIM homeobox genes in directing the dorsoventral trajectory of motor axons in the vertebrate limb. Cell. 2000;**102**(2):161-173. DOI: 10.1016/s0092-8674(00)00022-2

[40] Sockanathan S, Jessell TM. Motor neuron-derived retinoid signaling specifies the subtype identity of spinal motor neurons. Cell. 1998;**94**(4):503-514. DOI: 10.1016/s0092-8674(00)81591-3

[41] Tsuchida T, Ensini M, Morton SB, Baldassare M, Edlund T, Jessell TM, et al. Topographic organization of embryonic motor neurons defined by expression of LIM homeobox genes. Cell. 1994;**79**(6):957-970. DOI: 10.1016/0092-8674(94)90027-2

[42] Eberhart J, Swartz ME, Koblar SA, Pasquale EB, Krull CE. EphA4 constitutes a population-specific guidance cue for motor neurons. Developmental Biology. 2002;**247**(1):89-101. DOI: 10.1006/dbio.2002.0695

[43] Kania A, Jessell TM. Topographic motor projections in the limb imposed by LIM homeodomain protein regulation of ephrin-A:EphA interactions. Neuron. 2003;**38**(4):581-596. DOI: 10.1016/s0896-6273(03)00292-7

[44] Luria V, Krawchuk D, Jessell TM, Laufer E, Kania A. Specification of motor axon trajectory by ephrin-B: EphB signaling: Symmetrical control of axonal patterning in the developing limb. Neuron. 2008;**60**(6):1039-1053. DOI: 10.1016/j.neuron.2008.11.011

[45] Tiret L, Le Mouellic H, Maury M, Brûlet P. Increased apoptosis of motoneurons and altered somatotopic maps in the brachial spinal cord of Hoxc-8-deficient mice. Development. 1998;**125**(2):279-291. DOI: 10.1242/dev.125.2.279

[46] Catela C, Shin MM, Lee DH, Liu JP, Dasen JS. Hox proteins coordinate motor neuron differentiation and connectivity programs through ret/Gfrα genes. Cell Reports. 2016;**14**(8):1901-1915. DOI: 10.1016/j.celrep.2016.01.067. Epub 2016 Feb 18

[47] De Marco Garcia NV, Jessell TM. Early motor neuron pool identity and muscle nerve trajectory defined by postmitotic restrictions in Nkx6.1 activity. Neuron. 2008;**57**(2):217-231. DOI: 10.1016/j.neuron.2007.11.033

[48] Haase G, Dessaud E, Garcès A, de Bovis B, Birling M, Filippi P, et al. GDNF acts through PEA3 to regulate cell body positioning and muscle innervation of specific motor neuron pools. Neuron. 2002;**35**(5):893-905. DOI: 10.1016/s0896-6273(02)00864-4

[49] Zengel JE, Reid SA, Sypert GW, Munson JB. Membrane electrical properties and prediction of motor-unit type of medial gastrocnemius motoneurons in the cat. Journal of Neurophysiology. 1985;**53**(5):1323-1344. DOI: 10.1152/jn.1985.53.5.1323

[50] Kanning KC, Kaplan A, Henderson CE. Motor neuron diversity in development and disease. Annual Review of Neuroscience. 2010;**33**:409-440. DOI: 10.1146/annurev.neuro.051508.135722

[51] Burke RE, Levine DN, Tsairis P, Zajac FE 3rd. Physiological types and histochemical profiles in motor units of the cat gastrocnemius. The Journal of Physiology. 1973;**234**(3):723-748. DOI: 10.1113/jphysiol.1973.sp010369

[52] Burke RE, Rudomin P. Spinal nervous and synapses. In: Handbook of Physiology. The Nervous System. Cellular Biology of Neurons. Hoboken, New Jersey, USA: John Wiley & Sons, Inc.; 2011. DOI: 10.1002/cphy.cp010124

[53] Burke RE. Motor units: Anatomy, physiology, and functional organization. In: Handbook of Physiology, the Nervous System, Motor Control. Hoboken, New Jersey, USA: John Wiley & Sons, Inc.; 2011. DOI: 10.1002/cphy.cp010210

[54] Henneman E, Somjen G, Carpenter DO. Functional significance of

cell size inspinal motoneurons. Journal of Neurophysiology. 1965;**28**:560-580

[55] Henneman E, Somjen G, Carpenter D, O. Excitability and inhibitability of motoneurons of different sizes. Journal of Neurophysiology. 1965;**28**(3):599-620

[56] Burke RE. Motor unit types: Functional specializations in motor control. Trends in Neurosciences. 1980;**3**:255-258

[57] Heckman CJ, Johnson M, Mottram C, Schuster J. Persistent inward currents in spinal motoneurons and their influence on human motoneuron firing patterns. The Neuroscientist. 2008;**14**(3):264-275. DOI: 10.1177/1073858408314986. Epub 2008 Apr 1

[58] Kernell D. High frequency repetitive firing of cat lumbosacral motoneurones stimulated by long-lasting injected currents. Acta Physiologica Scandinavica. 1965;**65**:74-86. DOI: 10.1111/j.1748-1716.1965.tb04251.x

[59] Heckman CJ, Enoka RM. Physiology of the motor neuron and the motor unit. In: Clinical Neurophysiology of Motor Neuron Diseases Handbook of Clinical Neurophysiology. Vol. 4. Amsterdam, The Netherlands: Elsevier; 2004. DOI: 10.1016/S1567-4231(04)04006-7

[60] Binder MD, Heckman CJ, Powers RK. The physiological control of motor neuron activity. In: Comprehensive Physiology. Hoboken, New Jersey, USA: John Wiley & Sons, Inc.; 2011. DOI: 10.1002/cphy.cp120101

[61] Bakels R, Kernell D. Matching between motoneurone and muscle unit properties in rat medial gastrocnemius. The Journal of Physiology. 1993;**463**:307-324. DOI: 10.1113/jphysiol.1993.sp019596

[62] Gardiner PF. Physiological properties of motoneurons innervating different muscle unit types in rat gastrocnemius. Journal of Neurophysiology. 1993;**69**(4):1160-1170. DOI: 10.1152/jn.1993.69.4.1160

[63] Piehl F, Arvidsson U, Hökfelt T, Cullheim S. Calcitonin gene-related peptide-like immunoreactivity in motoneuron pools innervating different hind limb muscles in the rat. Experimental Brain Research. 1993;**96**(2):291-303. DOI: 10.1007/BF00227109

[64] Ringer C, Weihe E, Schütz B. Calcitonin gene-related peptide expression levels predict motor neuron vulnerability in the superoxide dismutase 1-G93A mouse model of amyotrophic lateral sclerosis. Neurobiology of Disease. 2012;**45**(1):547-554. DOI: 10.1016/j.nbd.2011.09.011. Epub 2011 Sep 21

[65] Enjin A, Rabe N, Nakanishi ST, Vallstedt A, Gezelius H, Memic F, et al. Identification of novel spinal cholinergic genetic subtypes disclose Chodl and Pitx2 as markers for fast motor neurons and partition cells. The Journal of Comparative Neurology. 2010;**518**(12):2284-2304. DOI: 10.1002/cne.22332

[66] Kaplan A, Spiller KJ, Towne C, Kanning KC, Choe GT, Geber A, et al. Neuronal matrix metalloproteinase-9 is a determinant of selective neurodegeneration. Neuron. 2014;**81**(2):333-348. DOI: 10.1016/j.neuron.2013.12.009

[67] Mueller D, Cherukuri P, Henningfeld K, Poh CH, Wittler L, Grote P, et al. Dlk1 promotes a fast motor neuron biophysical signature required for peak force execution. Science. 2014;**343**(6176):1264-1266. DOI: 10.1126/science.1246448

[68] Chakkalakal JV, Nishimune H, Ruas JL, Spiegelman BM, Sanes JR. Retrograde influence of muscle fibers on their innervation revealed by a novel marker for slow motoneurons. Development. 2010;**137**(20):3489-3499. DOI: 10.1242/dev.053348. Epub 2010 Sep 15

[69] Deardorff AS, Romer SH, Deng Z, Bullinger KL, Nardelli P, Cope TC, et al. Expression of postsynaptic Ca^{2+}-activated K^{+} (SK) channels at C-bouton synapses in mammalian lumbar-motoneurons. The Journal of Physiology. 2013;**591**(4):875-897. DOI: 10.1113/jphysiol.2012.240879. Epub 2012 Nov 5

[70] Shneider NA, Brown MN, Smith CA, Pickel J, Alvarez FJ. Gamma motor neurons express distinct genetic markers at birth and require muscle spindle-derived GDNF for postnatal survival. Neural Development. 2009;**4**:42. DOI: 10.1186/1749-8104-4-42

[71] Friese A, Kaltschmidt JA, Ladle DR, Sigrist M, Jessell TM, Arber S. Gamma and alpha motor neurons distinguished by expression of transcription factor Err3. Proceedings of the National Academy of Sciences of the United States of America. 2009;**106**(32):13588-13593. DOI: 10.1073/pnas.0906809106. Epub 2009 Jul 27

[72] Misawa H, Hara M, Tanabe S, Niikura M, Moriwaki Y, Okuda T. Osteopontin is an alpha motor neuron marker in the mouse spinal cord. Journal of Neuroscience Research. 2012;**90**(4):732-742. DOI: 10.1002/jnr.22813

[73] Edwards IJ, Bruce G, Lawrenson C, Howe L, Clapcote SJ, Deuchars SA, et al. Na+/K+ ATPase α1 and α3 isoforms are differentially expressed in α- and γ-motoneurons. The Journal of Neuroscience. 2013;**33**(24):9913-9919. DOI: 10.1523/JNEUROSCI.5584-12.2013

[74] Yasvoina MV, Genç B, Jara JH, Sheets PL, Quinlan KA, Milosevic A, et al. eGFP expression under UCHL1 promoter genetically labels corticospinal motor neurons and a subpopulation of degeneration-resistant spinal motor neurons in an ALS mouse model. The Journal of Neuroscience. 2013;**33**(18):7890-7904. DOI: 10.1523/JNEUROSCI.2787-12.2013

[75] Ruegsegger C, Maharjan N, Goswami A, Filézac de L'Etang A, Weis J, Troost D, et al. Aberrant association of misfolded SOD1 with Na(+)/K(+)ATPase-α3 impairs its activity and contributes to motor neuron vulnerability in ALS. Acta Neuropathologica. 2016;**131**(3):427-451. DOI: 10.1007/s00401-015-1510-4. Epub 2015 Nov 30

[76] Dobretsov M, Stimers JR. Neuronal function and alpha3 isoform of the Na/K-ATPase. Frontiers in Bioscience. 2005;**10**:2373-2396. DOI: 10.2741/1704

[77] Manuel M, Zytnicki D. Molecular and electrophysiological properties of mouse motoneuron and motor unit subtypes. Current Opinion in Physiology. 2019;**8**:23-29. DOI: 10.1016/j.cophys.2018.11.008. Epub 2018 Dec 1

[78] Bessou P, Emonet-Dénand F, Laporte Y. Motor fibres innervating extrafusal and intrafusal muscle fibres in the cat. The Journal of Physiology. 1965;**180**(3):649-672. DOI: 10.1113/jphysiol.1965.sp007722

[79] Hulliger M. The mammalian muscle spindle and its central control. Reviews of Physiology, Biochemistry and Pharmacology. 1984;**101**:1-110. DOI: 10.1007/BFb0027694

[80] Taylor A. Muscle receptors in the control of voluntary movement.

Paraplegia. 1972;**9**(4):167-172. DOI: 10.1038/sc.1971.28

[81] Fitz-Ritson D. The anatomy and physiology of the muscle spindle, and its role in posture and movement: A review. The Journal of the Canadian Chiropractic Association. 1982;**26**(4):144-150

[82] Kuffler SW, Hunt CC, Quilliam JP. Function of medullated small-nerve fibers in mammalian ventral roots; efferent muscle spindle innervation. Journal of Neurophysiology. 1951;**14**(1):29-54. DOI: 10.1152/jn.1951.14.1.29

[83] Hunt CC, Kuffler SW. Further study of efferent small-nerve fibers to mammalian muscle spindles; multiple spindle innervation and activity during contraction. The Journal of Physiology. 1951;**113**(2-3):283-297. DOI: 10.1113/jphysiol.1951.sp004572

[84] Eccles JC, Eccles RM, Iggo A, Lundberg A. Electrophysiological studies on gamma motoneurones. Acta Physiologica Scandinavica. 1960;**50**:32-40. DOI: 10.1111/j.1748-1716.1960.tb02070.x

[85] Kemm RE, Westbury DR. Some properties of spinal gamma-motoneurones in the cat, determined by micro-electrode recording. The Journal of Physiology. 1978;**282**:59-71. DOI: 10.1113/jphysiol.1978.sp012448

[86] Matthews PB. The differentiation of two types of fusimotor fibre by their effects on the dynamic response of muscle spindle primary endings. Quarterly Journal of Experimental Physiology and Cognate Medical Sciences. 1962;**47**:324-333

[87] Enjin A, Leão KE, Mikulovic S, Le Merre P, Tourtellotte WG, Kullander K. Sensorimotor function is modulated by the serotonin receptor 1d, a novel marker for gamma motor neurons. Molecular and Cellular Neurosciences. 2012;**49**(3):322-332. DOI: 10.1016/j.mcn.2012.01.003. Epub 2012 Jan 17

[88] Khan MN, Cherukuri P, Negro F, Rajput A, Fabrowski P, Bansal V, et al. ERR2 and ERR3 promote the development of gamma motor neuron functional properties required for proprioceptive movement control. PLoS Biology. 2022;**20**(12):e3001923. DOI: 10.1371/journal.pbio.3001923

[89] Leksell L. The action potentials and excitatory effects of the small ventral root fibres to skeletal muscle. Acta Physiologica Scandinavica. 1945;**10**(1(Suppl. 31)):1-84

[90] Katz B. The efferent regulation of the muscle spindle in the frog. The Journal of Experimental Biology. 1949;**26**(2):201-217. DOI: 10.1242/jeb.26.2.201

[91] Henneman E. Relation between size of neurons and their susceptibility to discharge. Science. 1957;**126**(3287):1345-1347. DOI: 10.1126/science.126.3287.1345

[92] Ellaway PH, Taylor A, Durbaba R. Muscle spindle and fusimotor activity in locomotion. Journal of Anatomy. 2015;**227**(2):157-166. DOI: 10.1111/joa.12299. Epub 2015 Jun 5

[93] Bessou P, Emonet-Denand F, Laporte Y. Occurrence of intrafusal muscle fibres innervation by branches of slow α motor fibres in the cat. Nature. 1963;**198**(4880):594-595

[94] Kernell D. Input resistance, electrical excitability, and size of ventral horn cells in cat spinal cord. Science. 1966;**152**(3729):1637-1640. DOI: 10.1126/science.152.3729.1637

[95] Kelley KW, Ben Haim L, Schirmer L, Tyzack GE, Tolman M, Miller JG, et al. Kir4.1-dependent astrocyte-fast motor neuron interactions are required for peak strength. Neuron. 2018;**98**(2):306-319.e7. DOI: 10.1016/j.neuron.2018.03.010. Epub 2018 Apr 5

[96] D'Elia KP, Hameedy H, Goldblatt D, Frazel P, Kriese M, Zhu Y, et al. Determinants of motor neuron functional subtypes important for locomotor speed. Cell Reports. 2023;**42**(9):113049. DOI: 10.1016/j.celrep.2023.113049. Epub ahead of print

[97] Patel T, Hammelman J, Aziz S, et al. Transcriptional dynamics of murine motor neuron maturation *in vivo* and *in vitro*. Nature Communications. 2022;**13**:5427. DOI: 10.1038/s41467-022-33022-4

[98] Hobert O, Kratsios P. Neuronal identity control by terminal selectors in worms, flies, and chordates. Current Opinion in Neurobiology. 2019;**56**:97-105. DOI: 10.1016/j.conb.2018.12.006. Epub 2019 Jan 18

[99] Barker D. The morphology of muscle receptors. In: Hunt CC, editor. Handbook of Sensory Physiology Vol. III/2, Muscle Receptors. Berlin-Heidelberg-New York: Springer-Verlag; 1974

[100] Goody MF, Carter EV, Kilroy EA, Maves L, Henry CA. "muscling" throughout life: Integrating studies of muscle development, homeostasis, and disease in zebrafish. Current Topics in Developmental Biology. 2017;**124**:197-234. DOI: 10.1016/bs.ctdb.2016.11.002. Epub 2016 Dec 23

[101] Ampatzis K, Song J, Ausborn J, El Manira A. Pattern of innervation and recruitment of different classes of motoneurons in adult zebrafish. The Journal of Neuroscience. 2013;**33**(26):10875-10886. DOI: 10.1523/JNEUROSCI.0896-13.2013

[102] Ampatzis K, Song J, Ausborn J, El Manira A. Separate microcircuit modules of distinct v2a interneurons and motoneurons control the speed of locomotion. Neuron. 2014;**83**(4):934-943. DOI: 10.1016/j.neuron.2014.07.018. Epub 2014 Aug 7

[103] Gabriel JP, Ausborn J, Ampatzis K, Mahmood R, Eklöf-Ljunggren E, El Manira A. Principles governing recruitment of motoneurons during swimming in zebrafish. Nature Neuroscience. 2011;**14**(1):93-99. DOI: 10.1038/nn.2704. Epub 2010 Nov 28

[104] Armstrong RB, Phelps RO. Muscle fiber type composition of the rat hindlimb. The American Journal of Anatomy. 1984;**171**(3):259-272. DOI: 10.1002/aja.1001710303

[105] Maeda N, Miyoshi S, Toh H. First observation of a muscle spindle in fish. Nature. 1983;**302**(5903):61-62. DOI: 10.1038/302061a0

Chapter 3

Exploring the Potential for Biomaterials to Improve the Development of Spinal Motor Neurons from Induced Pluripotent Stem Cells

Juyoung Seong, Changho Chun, Alec S.T. Smith, Jinmyoung Joo and David L. Mack

Abstract

Neuromuscular diseases (NMDs) are primarily caused by progressive degeneration of motor neurons that leads to skeletal muscle denervation. The physiological complexity and cellular heterogeneity of individual motor units make understanding the underlying pathological mechanisms of NMDs difficult. Moreover, the demonstrable species specificity of neuromuscular synapse structure and function underscores the need to develop reliable human models of neuromuscular physiology with which to study disease etiology and test the efficacy of novel therapeutics. In this regard, human-induced pluripotent stem cells (hiPSCs) represent a valuable tool for developing such models. However, the lack of cellular diversity and transcriptomic immaturity of motor neurons derived from iPSCs has so far limited their downstream applications. To address this shortcoming, biomaterials such as 3D biopolymer scaffolds and biocompatible nanoparticles have been investigated for their ability to improve current neuronal differentiation protocols. In this review, we summarize current efforts and limitations associated with the use of functional biomaterials to increase the physiological relevance of stem cell-derived motor neurons. We also suggest potential future directions for research using biomaterials to overcome outstanding issues related to stem cell-based neuromuscular tissue production for use in NMD modeling applications.

Keywords: pluripotent stem cell, motor neuron differentiation, biomaterials, scaffolds, nanoparticles

1. Introduction

Neuromuscular diseases (NMDs) refer to a set of conditions that affect motor units, which are functional units comprising individual spinal motor neurons, their axons, the axon's terminal nerve branches, neuromuscular junctions (NMJ), and the skeletal muscle fibers connected to these junctions (**Figure 1**). One of the most the well-known NMDs is amyotrophic lateral sclerosis (ALS) (**Figure 2**). ALS is a neurodegenerative disorder characterized by the degeneration of upper and lower motor neurons, leading to a progressive loss of motor function and ultimately resulting in death, often due to respiratory failure [1, 2]. Unfortunately, the disease is generally fatal within 3 to 5 years after diagnosis [3]. It typically appears in mid-adulthood, with the average age of onset being 55 years, although it can begin as early as the first or second decade of life or even develop later in life [4, 5]. ALS has an annual diagnosis rate of 1–2 individuals per 100,000 in most countries [1, 2]. In the United States and the United Kingdom, ALS is responsible for more than 1 in 500 deaths in adults, indicating that over 15 million people currently alive may eventually succumb to this disease [1]. Another significant motor neuron disease that is typically classified as an NMD is spinal muscular atrophy (SMA). The global occurrence of SMA is approximately 1 in 40–60 [6, 7]. SMA involves the disruption of the motor unit, leading to the degeneration of proximal motor axons, loss of synaptic inputs to cell bodies, and, ultimately, the death of motor neuron cell bodies [6].

ALS and SMA share a common symptom, and current approaches to managing these NMDs is centered around addressing symptoms, such as preserving weakened muscle function, rather than tackling the root cause of the disease. The paucity of effective treatments for NMDs such as ALS and SMA has led to a recent effort to develop more predictive preclinical models with which to model these conditions and evaluate novel therapeutic efficacy.

Historically, the *in vitro* study of motor neurons has relied on sourcing cells from spinal cord tissue derived from embryonic chicks and rodents [8–14]. Such neurons are more similar to human cells than to worm-like animals and arthropods, but they still have different developmental patterns and morphologies compared to humans, particularly in the distribution of motor nerve terminals and their size and conformation [15]. Animal models are the current "gold standard" preclinical method for

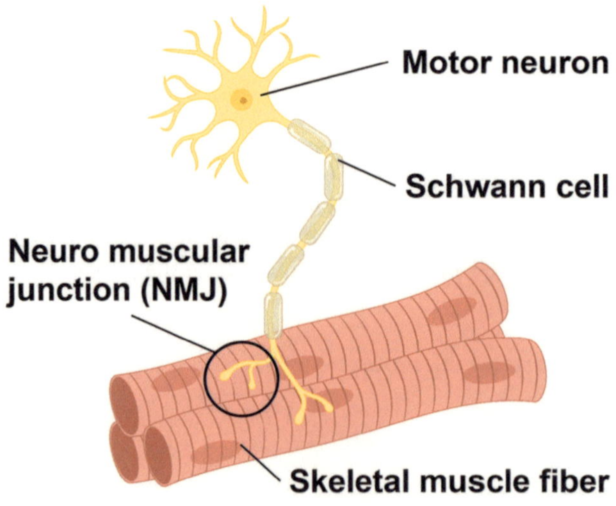

Figure 1.
Motor unit. Motor units are composed of lower motor neurons, neuromuscular junctions (NMJs), and skeletal muscle fiber.

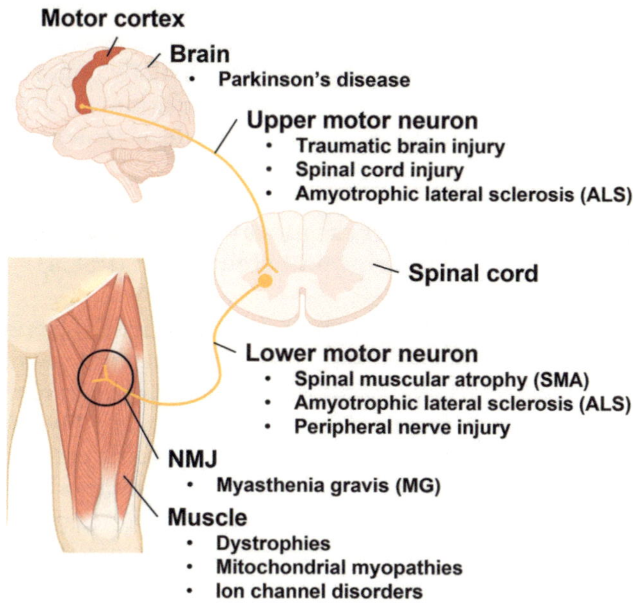

Figure 2.
Neuromuscular disease (NMD). NMDs encompass cellular disorders of the motor unit. Each unique disorder affects different aspect of the motor unit.

evaluating the efficacy of novel ALS therapeutics. However, the last 20 years have seen rigorous animal tests on multiple ALS-targeted drugs that prolonged life in the animal but failed to elicit a therapeutic benefit in humans [16]. This has fueled a recent interest in developing alternative, human-based preclinical assays to better inform patient responses to compound exposure. The establishment of such assays is dependent on the establishment of robust models of human motor neurons.

To address this need, researchers have turned to human-induced pluripotent stem cell (iPSC) technology to derive motor neurons that more accurately reflect the cells present in patients. The advantage of human iPSC-derived motor neurons is that they have unlimited expansion potential and can generate large homogeneous populations of neurons for downstream studies. This makes them suitable for studies requiring a large number of neurons for repetitive tasks, such as drug screening, proteomics, and biochemistry [17]. Additionally, human iPSC-derived motor neurons retain patient-specific gene mutations, making it possible to study individual patient genotype–phenotype relationships *in vitro* [18].

Despite those efforts, a significant challenge in using human iPSC-derived motor neurons is their relative immaturity compared to primary motor neurons. This is because the culture process typically used to differentiate human iPSCs into motor neurons does not encapsulate the complexity of the developing spinal cord *in vivo* and is conducted on a timescale (days to weeks) that is far more rapid than native embryogenesis and subsequent postnatal development (months to years). As such, some concerns remain that human iPSC-derived motor neurons may not exhibit all of the same physiological properties as primary motor neurons.

As a result, it is essential to improve the maturity of human iPSC-derived motor neurons to increase their suitability for use in next-generation disease modeling and/or drug screening applications. This maturation process is crucial for ensuring that the findings obtained using human iPSC-derived motor neurons are reliable and accurately represent the relevant biological processes as they occur *in vivo*. Achieving more mature cultured human motor neurons is particularly important to the endeavors to model NMDs such as ALS that exhibit symptomatic onset at stages of life that are far later than embryogenesis and early postnatal development.

2. Unaddressed problems in current motor neuron differentiation strategies using induced pluripotent stem cells (iPSCs)

The development of induced pluripotent stem cells (iPSCs) has enabled researchers to study many *human diseases,* including congenital neurodegenerative diseases, from a developmental perspective. Established somatic reprogramming techniques, using only four transcription factors (Oct4, Sox2, Klf4, and c-Myc), enable scientist to generate patient-derived stem cell lines harboring specific patient mutations. Advances in genetic editing strategies have also facilitated the establishment of isogenic controls from these mutants and comparison of cells derived from these paired iPSC population allow analysis of how a specific patient mutation alters the phenotype of cells that otherwise harbor identical genotypes [19]. Despite their enormous potential to replace or augment animal disease models, current neuronal iPSC models come with critical shortcomings that have been a major roadblock for their wider adoption in biomedical applications. Although iPSCs show similar transcriptomic profiles with those of embryonic stem cells (ESC), especially for the genes governing pluripotency, even state-of-the-art differentiation strategies for generating human neurons from iPSCs are far from perfect in terms of their capacity to produce cells that accurately reflect their *in vivo* counterparts [20–23]. Populations obtained from 20 to 50 days of *in vitro* neuronal differentiation often contain a mixture of various unknown subtypes of neurons, and glial cells. Even cells from outside the neuroglial lineage are often observed, and these cells tend to outcompete the postmitotic neuronal populations over time [22–25]. Moreover, commonly used differentiation protocols often lack reproducibility, which can result in the production of transcriptionally and functionally inconsistent neuronal populations from one batch to the next. Thus, it is reasonable to posit that such shortcomings in iPSC differentiation methods will have a negative impact on the accuracy and reproducibility of downstream research results when iPSC-derived neurons are used as predictors of human neural responses to chemical or pathological challenges. In addition to the disparity between *in vivo* human neurons and iPSC-derived neurons, a more challenging issue lies in the fact that we do not know how to reliably promote the maturation of iPSC-derived neurons toward an adult phenotype, which is critical for the study of late-onset neurodegenerative disorders such as ALS and Parkinson's disease (PD) [18, 26–30].

Most current motor neuron differentiation protocols rely on small molecule treatments to sequentially induce ectoderm, neuroectoderm, ventral spinal neuron progenitors, and finally a mixture of premature motor neurons and interneurons. This is often then followed by treatment with trophic factors to induce further maturation of those early-stage neurons [31–34]. In the majority of these protocols, undifferentiated iPSCs are initially treated with dual-SMAD inhibitors (SB431542 and LDN193189) to inhibit TGF-beta and BMP signaling pathways, which drives pluripotent stem cells toward the ectoderm lineage. Du *et al*. found that additional treatment of CHIR99021, which turns on the Wnt pathway, significantly enriches early-stage cultures with proliferative neural progenitors and this, in turn, results in the formation of a greater number of so-called "neural rosettes" around 10 days post-induction. A critically important small molecule that most protocols use to provide a caudalization cue to the developing neural progenitors is retinoic acid (RA) [35]. RA is a pivotal molecule regulating embryonic patterning and development. It is a metabolic product of vitamin A (retinol) synthesized by the paraxial mesoderm. RA mediates the expression of HOX genes that are sequentially activated during embryonic development and is responsible for regulating the regional patterning of neuronal subtypes vertically along the spinal cord (**Figure 3**). The timing of RA expression dictates when colinear HOX gene expression is stopped, thereby controlling the regional patterning of neurons as well as promoting the transition from neuromesoderm into neuroectoderm [36, 37]. Given the importance of RA physiology in spinal motor neuron development, it has been a major target of research to improve motor neuron differentiation protocols. However, our understanding of RA-mediated motor neuron differentiation has not progressed far beyond the initial findings regarding limited aspects of its mechanism of action, leaving an important knowledge gap in terms of our understanding of spinal motor neuron development.

Once a caudal phenotype is established by RA, sonic hedgehog (SHH) or its agonist (e.g., purmorphamine with or without SAG (Smo agonist) supplementation) is then typically used to derive progenitors toward a ventral spinal identity. SHH is a vertebrate homolog of the Drosophila protein hedgehog and is expressed by the

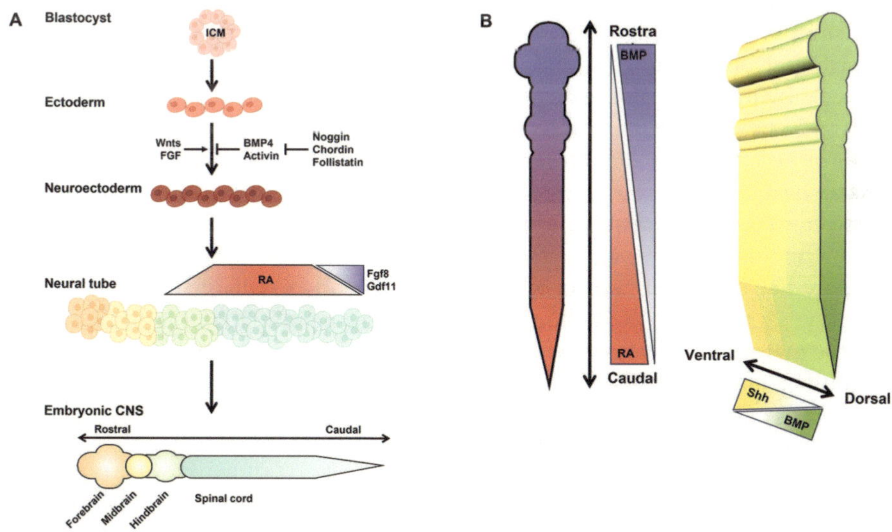

Figure 3.
Schematic illustration of the spinal cord development in vivo. (A) In the early stages of development, a process called gastrulation occurs, which leads to the differentiation of cells in the inner cell mass (ICM) into three germ layers: Ectoderm, endoderm, and mesoderm. The dorsal part of the ectoderm undergoes further specialization into the neuroectoderm by inhibiting BMP and activin signaling while enhancing FGF and Wnt signaling, particularly in higher organisms. Neuralization progresses as a neural plate form and subsequently folds to create neural folds, which then fuse to form the neural tube. The neural tube is organized along the anterior-posterior axis (rostral-caudal) through the presence of a retinoic acid (RA) gradient, primarily regulated by Raldh2. RA plays a crucial role in establishing the initial boundaries between the spinal cord and hindbrain versus forebrain and hindbrain. Fgfs and Gdf11 counteract the effects of RA and contribute to the specification of more caudal spinal cord cell types. (B) the schematic illustrates key signaling factors that play a crucial role in organizing the anterior–posterior (rostral–caudal) and dorsal–ventral axes of the developing nervous system during embryonic development. It specifically focuses on a coronal section through the developing telencephalon. (fibroblast growth factor: FGF, bone morphogenetic protein: BMP, retinoic acid: RA, sonic hedgehog: Shh).

notochord and floor plate in the developing spinal cord. It provides signals necessary for positional patterning in the spinal cord. The concentration gradient of SHH determines whether the unpatterned progenitor cells have dorsal or ventral identity during the course of spinal neuron development. Despite the present understanding and detailed knowledge on the spinal neuron development and the cues necessary to drive the adoption of a motor neuron phenotype, the cells obtained from these protocols typically result in the adoption of an embryonic or neonatal phenotype. The use of particular biomaterials that exhibit various functionality upon applications is one of the promising strategic methods to achieve greater levels of maturation in these cells *in vitro*. Motor neuron differentiation of iPSCs using such functional biomaterials to improve the physiological relevance *in vitro* culture is discussed in detail below.

3. The use of biomaterials to improve the physiological relevance of iPSC-derived human neurons

Variety of biomaterials, as forms of hydrogels, nanoparticles, scaffolds and mesh, and so forth, have been recognized as attractive resources in the field of regenerative medicine and tissue engineering due to their physical and chemical tunability as well as their biocompatibility with most human stem cells (**Figure 4**). In particular, the development of biocompatible materials that can support functional tissue generation has gained significant interest in recent years.

For example, a hydrogel is a hydrophilic polymer resembling human tissue with high biocompatibility. Various monomeric compounds have been studied to form the hydrogel by modulating the degree of cross-linking to control the mechanical strength and releasing kinetics of embedded payloads such as growth factors [38]. Gelatin is one of the natural polymers that is a precursor of collagen. Both collagen and gelatin have high biocompatibility and low toxicity, but there are some issues regarding complex purification and modifying short degradation rates [39]. Both of them are often used to form an extracellular matrix (ECM). Also, serum albumin is a natural polymer used to construct ECM [40]. It has long a half-life compared to other natural polymers [40–42]. A carbon nanotube is also used to make ECM because it is a tunable material that possesses mechanical and electrical properies [43] and it is easy to modify its surface. Moreover, it has biocompatibility and high cell attachment. Those features can be adjusted to mimic ECM.

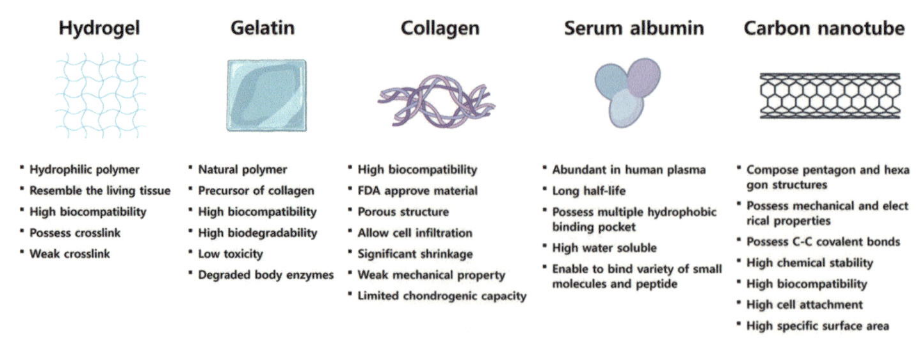

Figure 4.
Characteristics of biomaterials in scaffolds. Each class of biomaterials has numerous advantages and disadvantages in terms of its suitability as an engineered neural scaffold.

In addition to synthetic biomaterials, such as polyethylene glycol (PEG), polylactide-co-glycolic acid (PLGA) has been widely demonstrated to stem cell differentiation and tissue regeneration because of its tunable physical and chemical properties that provide beneficial effects to construct functional human tissues *in vivo*. The central hypothesis of applying such biomaterials to neural tissue engineering is that the physiological relevance of differentiating neurons will be readily improved by providing an extracellular microenvironment that more closely recapitulates the native spatiotemporal niche where these cells occupy in developing embryos. Specifically, researchers have attempted to recapitulate the extracellular microenvironment during neural development by taking into account factors such as the cell–matrix interaction, intracellular interactions within the given environment, the physical and mechanical characteristics of the matrix surrounding the neural tube, the topographical status of extracellular proteins, and the oxygen and nutrient provision capabilities of the matrix. In the following section, we summarized the advances and limitations of the biomaterials that have been used so far to recreate the surrounding environment of nervous tissue during the developmental stages. 3D scaffolds are widely used as a means of structural cues that are responsible for physical and mechanical properties of tissue microenvironment such as matrix stiffness, adhesion, and migration during neuronal differentiation. On the other hand, micro- and nanoparticles are utilized to control the biological cues through spatiotemporal release of active ingredients to differentiate the neurons. Importantly, we discuss ideas that may help to recapitulate the two critical characteristics of native spinal cord development: (1) the exquisite spatiotemporal control of inductive cues secreted around the neural tube, which are the main drivers of neuronal differentiation and specialization throughout the course of normal spinal cord development and (2) the dramatic conversion from flattened neural plate to 3D neural tube during early phases of spinal cord development. We believe that these issues constitute a root cause of the disparity between spinal neurons developed *in vitro* versus *in vivo*, and addressing these issues may help disentangle the remaining issues still plaguing iPSC-derived neuronal development *in vitro*.

4. 3D scaffolds: providing structural cues to iPSCs differentiation neurons

Conventional cell culture experiments, conducted on flat plastic surfaces, have provided us with a wealth of basic cell biology knowledge for decades. However, 2D culture schemes do not accurately recreate the physical cues, such as matrix stiffness, topology, and interaction between cells and matrix, which are present in the extracellular environment during native 3D tissue development *in vivo*. Additionally, neural differentiation on 2D surfaces often suffers from issues caused by neural sheet delamination, which results in poor longevity of cultured cell populations and batch-to-batch inconsistencies in differentiated populations. This becomes even more of a critical issue when it comes to generating multicellular tissues such as spinal cord that are required to have a continuous intracellular interactions and consistent delivery of differentiating cues from the surrounding microenvironments [44]. To address this issue, various biomaterials have been used to generate 3D scaffolds that provide a physiologically similar, material-permeable environment for exchanging morphogens, oxygen, and nutrients essential for each step of tissue development. Moreover, many studies have shown that 3D scaffold-mediated neural differentiation enables more complex interactions to develop between neural precursors and between cells and ECM proteins. Furthermore, such scaffolds provide better spatial organization of cells, which mimics the native environment during neurogenesis more closely.

Scaffolds can come in various shapes and geometries, such as fibrillar morphologies (3D structures composed of long, fibrous protein chains) with respect to length, thickness, surface structure (smooth vs. rugged), and overall shape (straight vs. curly), which can be modified to impact cell-to-cell and cell-to-matrix interactions. There are three categories of scaffolds to address the structural cues: surface property, mechanical property, and electrical property (**Table 1**). The surface properties of scaffolds can often be changed by modulating pH or using surfactants to affect material properties such as water uptake, compressive moduli, and cross-linking.

Category	Biomaterials	Cell	Effect	Ref.
Surface property	Hydrogel	ESC	Rough surface → Neuronal differentiation↑, viability↑	[45]
	Carbon nanotube	hNSC	Polarize surface → Axon growth↑	[46]
	Gold	Primary neuron	Increase anchoring sites → Neurites growth↑	[47]
Mechanical property	Hydrogel	NSC	Encapsulating cell → Neuronal differentiation↑, cell align↑	[48]
	Hydrogel	iPSC	Mimic ECM (change cross link) → Neuronal differentiation↑	[49]
	Gelatin	NSC	Mimic ECM (porous scaffold) → Infiltration of macrophage, microglia↓, Axonal regeneration, outgrowth↑	[50]
	Silica	NSC	Mimic ECM (various size of space) → Deliver amount↑	[51]
	Collagen	NSC	Mimic ECM (porous structure) → Neuron's functional maturity↑	[52]
	Gelatin hydrogel	Neuroblastoma cell	Surface modification + release RA → RA binding affinity↑ → Neuronal differentiation↑	[53]
	Serum albumin	hiPSC	Surface modification + release FGF2 → FGF2 binding affinity↑ → Neuronal differentiation↑ Neuronal maturation level↑	[42]
	Gelatin	NSC	Surface modification + release Neurotrophin3 → Neurotrophin3 binding affinity↑ → Neuronal differentiation ↑ Synapse formation↑	[50]
Electrical property	Serum albumin + Iron	hiPSC	Confer conductivity → Neuronal differentiation↑ Axon branches↑	[42]

Table 1.
Structural cues derived by 3D scaffolds used in neuronal differentiation.

Modulation of any of these properties could potentially affect the modality of neural differentiation within such structures. Therefore, it has been important to find a scaffold condition that promotes neurodevelopment that includes robust formation of axons and dendrites as well as the expression of neuron-specific proteins for synaptic transmission and electrophysiological function.

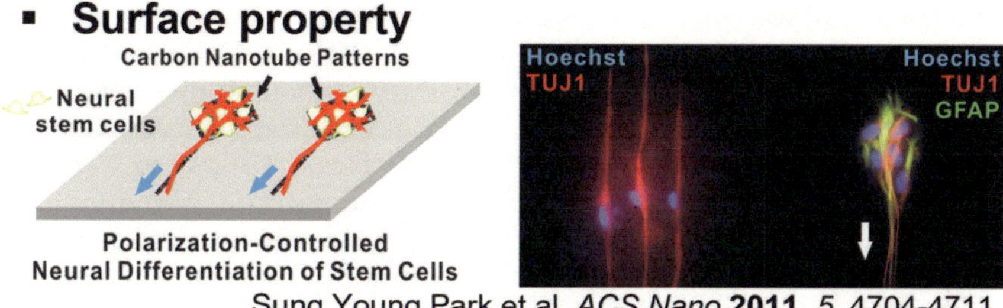

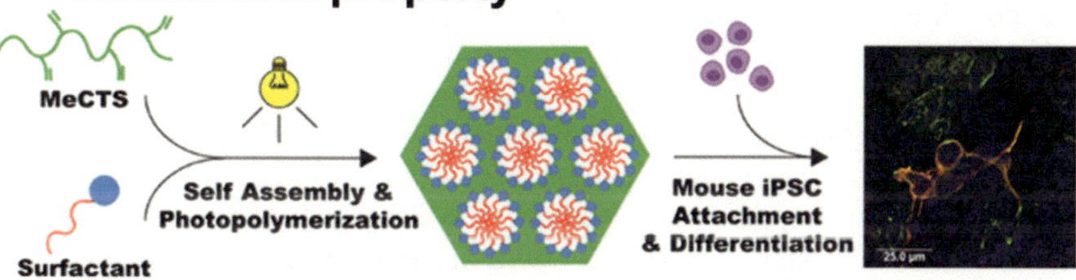

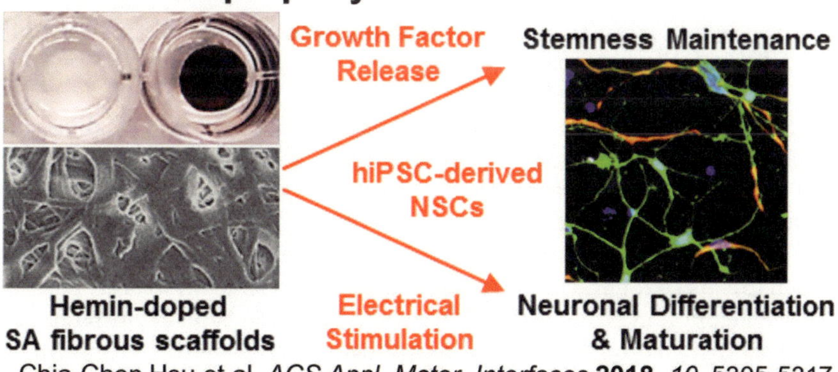

Figure 5.
Currently studied applications of scaffolds in neuronal differentiation. (A) An example of surface property modulation. Carbon nanotube (CNT) network patterns are utilized to achieve selective growth and polarization-controlled neuronal differentiation of human neural stem cells (hNSCs). CNT roughness promotes the adhesion and longevity of primary neurons. This CNT pattern induces the selective growth and differentiation of hNMSs. Also, the CNT pattern is able to maintain cell-to-cell interaction well. As a result, the CNT pattern is a more stable and versatile platform, with optimal nano-topography and biocompatibility, with which to regulate hNSC growth in vitro [46]. (B) An example of mechanical property modification. Surfactant templating is shown to effectively tune the water uptake and compressive modulus of photo-cross-linked chitosan hydrogels, mitigating property fluctuations with changing pH, enabling greater attachment of iPSCs, and enhancing neuronal differentiation [49]. (C) An example of electrical property modulation. Conductive scaffolds incorporating topographical, biochemical, and electrical stimuli support attachment, proliferation, neuronal differentiation, and maturation of iPSCs, demonstrating their potential for nerve regeneration strategies without the need for growth factor supplementation [42].

For the use of biomaterials in neural tissue generation and remodeling, there are preconditions to be satisfied. Scaffolds should have the ability to provide structural support that is tailored to the needs of the embedded stem cells (in terms of stiffness etc.) and provide correct guidance cues to the developing neurons by allowing small molecules in the medium to reach the entire population of cells at desired concentrations and kinetics during tissue formation. Although challenging, researchers have been trying to achieve this goal by modulating the structural parameters of scaffolds such as the pore size, porosity (% of void area relative to the entire surface area of the scaffold), and surface stiffness. Additionally, work has been performed that explores the binding of functional groups on to the scaffold surface to induce biochemical interactions between the matrix and the embedded cells [54, 55]. For example, adjusting surface stiffness and wettability have been shown to impact the number of neurites growing out of individual cells and the number of neuritic branches that develop from these projections, which are both major metrics for assessing neuronal differentiation and maturation in culture (**Figure** 5) [46, 52, 53, 56, 57]. The mechanical properties of the substrate and the interaction between the matrix structure and cells are also important factors to consider [40, 58–62]. Nanocomposite materials composed of synthetic polymers and fillers allow bulk and local modulation of physical properties to create a high surface area to volume ratio and control interfacial binding strength, which can enable the release of neurotrophic factors that induce neuronal differentiation [62–65]. Lastly, electrical properties of the scaffold, such as conductive nanostructures like silver, gold, and carbon, can affect cell adhesion, migration, and orientation by electrical stimulation, which can also impact neuronal differentiation [62, 66, 67].

5. Nanoparticles: controlling the spatiotemporal supplement of biological cues to iPSCs differentiation to neurons

In addition to the provision of structural guidance using biomaterial-based scaffolds, exposing developing stem cells to molecular cues in a spatiotemporally-controlled manner is another factor that is crucial to establish the mature neurons when attempting to recapitulate the native morphogen supply that is achieved during native spinal cord development. To this end, understanding the molecular supply mechanisms that determine spinal neuron cell fate is important. During spinal cord development, stem cells differentiate into each type of spinal neuron through the exquisite control of several morphogens and growth factors, which creates combinatorial gradients of factors releasing mainly from the notochord and paraxial mesoderm. However, *in vitro* differentiation schemes lack accuracy in terms of recreating these morphogen gradients, resulting in the formation of an often poorly defined population of neurons and glia at the end of the protocol. The lack of materials to function as a source of controlled morphogen release has been a major reason for this shortcoming in current protocols, exacerbated by our insufficient understanding of native morphogen supply scheme during spinal cord development. Therefore, there is an urgent need to develop material tools, with high cytocompatibility, to more closely mimic the exquisite biomolecule release schemes that exist *in vivo* and to do so in a tunable manner to be enable optimization of release kinetics for the various factors necessary to induce motor neuron differentiation (e.g., RA, SHH, SAG, etc.).

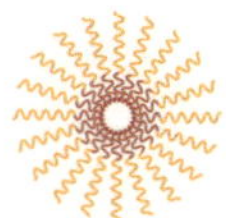

Polymer nanoparticle
Control the release by pH
High biocompatibility
Adjust surface modification
Self-aggregation
e.g. PEI, PLGA. etc

Inorganic nanoparticle
Porous structure
Tunable pore and particle size
Flexible payload
High biocompatibility
Strong stability
Potential toxicity
e.g MSN, IONP etc

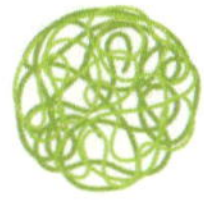

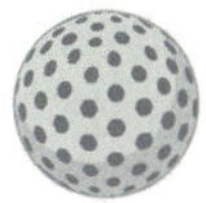

Figure 6.
Characteristics of nanoparticles for use as morphogen carriers. Each class of nanoparticle has numerous advantages and disadvantages regarding cargo and delivery. (poly(lactic-co-glycolic acid): PLGA, Polyethyleminine: PEI, mesoporous silica nanoparticle: MSN, iron oxide nanoparticle: IONP).

Nanoparticles are an attractive candidate to fulfill this requirement. Depending on the type of nanoparticle, its surface can be modified for active targeting, penetrating barriers, and releasing molecules through pH-responsive properties while also avoiding clearance by the immune system [68–71]. To improve neuronal differentiation, researchers have been developing many different types of nanoparticle carriers, such as DNA nanostructures, mesoporous silica nanoparticles (MSN), and polyethyleneimine (PEI) to effectively deliver neurogenic-inductive factors such as signaling ligands, DNA, siRNA, and mRNA into early-stage differentiating neuronal progenitors (**Figure 6**). In the context of supporting controlled release of morphogens, a study demonstrated that morphogen-loaded nanoparticles could be used as a source of controlled molecule release to provide pivotal molecules for neurogenesis, such as RA. Since RA has a very short half-life (14 minutes in PBS), it is difficult to maintain its active form to induce an effective role for a long-term period of culture *in vitro*. Using nanoparticles to release RA can facilitate the conversion of stem cells into neural cells by activating neural signaling pathways and minimizing cell cytotoxicity

Materials	Cell	Cargo	Loading method	Ref.
TDN	NSC	DNA	Self-assembly	[72]
MOF	NSC	RA	Capillary action	[73]
MSN	ESC	RA	Electrostatic interaction	[74]
PEI	ESC	RA	Electrostatic interaction	[75]
PEI	SVZ	RA	Electrostatic interaction	[69]
PEI	SVZ	RA	Electrostatic interaction	[76]

(Tetrahedral DNA nanostructure: TDN, Metal-organic framework: MOF, Mesoporous silica nanoparticle: MSN, Polyethyleminine: PEI).

Table 2.
Nanoparticle used in neuronal differentiation.

(**Table 2**) [69, 73–76]. Such studies demonstrate that nanoparticles have a significant impact on neuronal differentiation from stem cell sources and with minimal effect on cell viability and proliferation. Nanoparticle modification can also provide an intracellular docking system for the simultaneous delivery of multiple factors to facilitate neuronal differentiation (**Figures 7–10**).

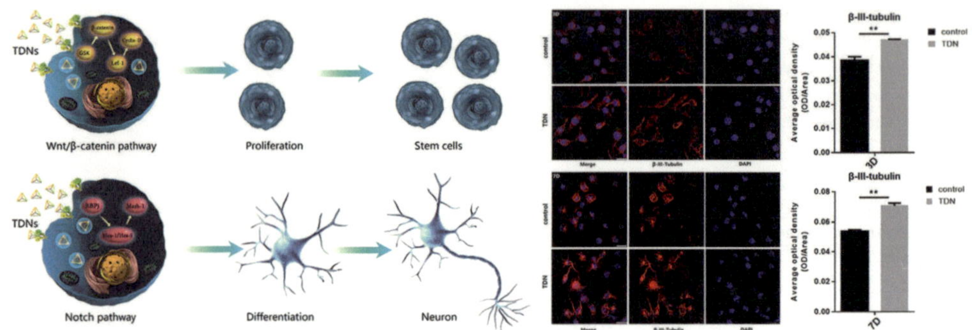

Figure 7.
Application of nanoparticle for neuronal differentiation: Tetrahedral DNA nanostructure (TDN). The study investigated the effects of TDN on neural stem cells, demonstrating that TDNs promote self-renewal through the Wnt/β-catenin pathway and enhance neuronal differentiation by inhibiting the notch signaling pathway and suggesting their potential for nerve tissue regeneration. Because using TDN increase uptake of cells in stem cells [72].

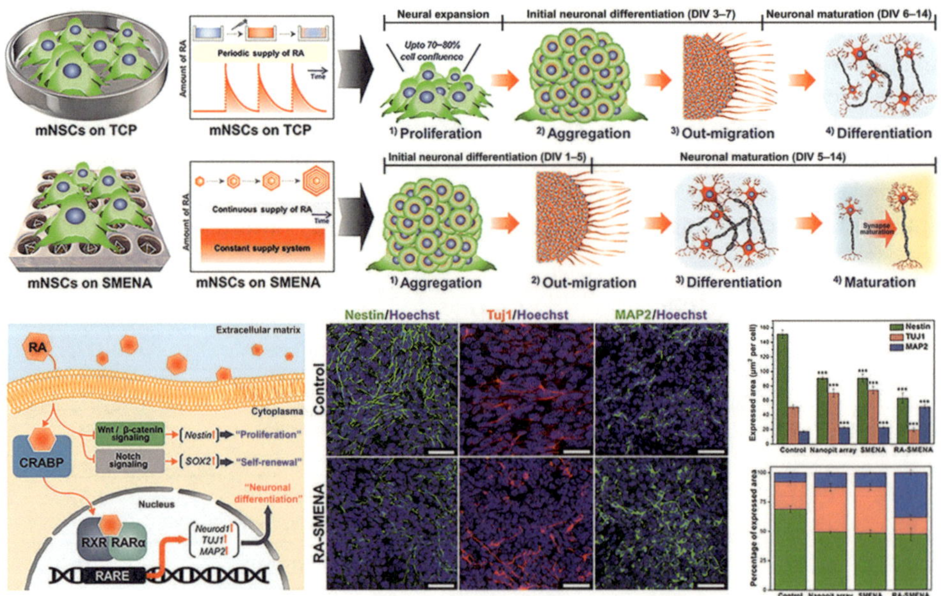

Figure 8.
Application of nanoparticle for neuronal differentiation: Metal-organic framework (MOF). The study introduces a new platform, called SMENA, which utilizes MOF-embedded nanopit arrays to provide a stable and continuous supply of retinoic acid, promoting enhanced neuronal cell generation and demonstrating potential for various stem cell-based regenerative therapies [73].

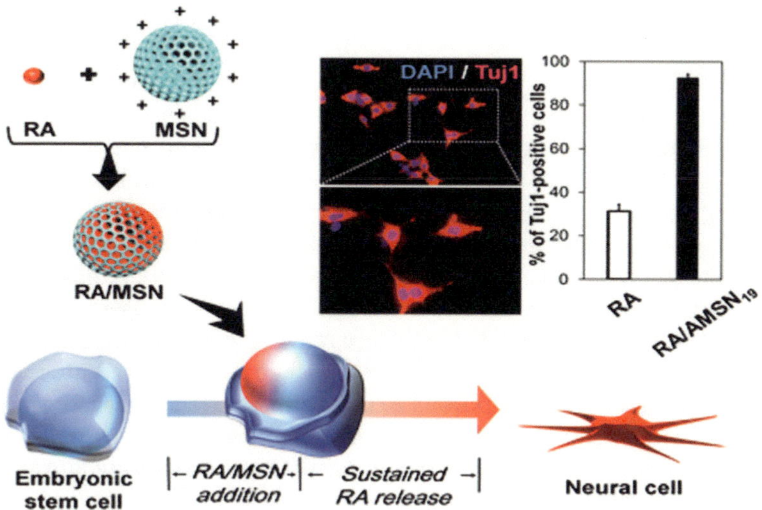

Figure 9.
Applications of nanoparticle for neuronal differentiation: Mesoporous silica nanoparticle. This study used MSN as a delivery carrier of RA, which enabled rapid and high-quality neural differentiation of mouse embryonic stem cells, resulting in the successful derivation of stable neurite marker-expressing neural cells [74].

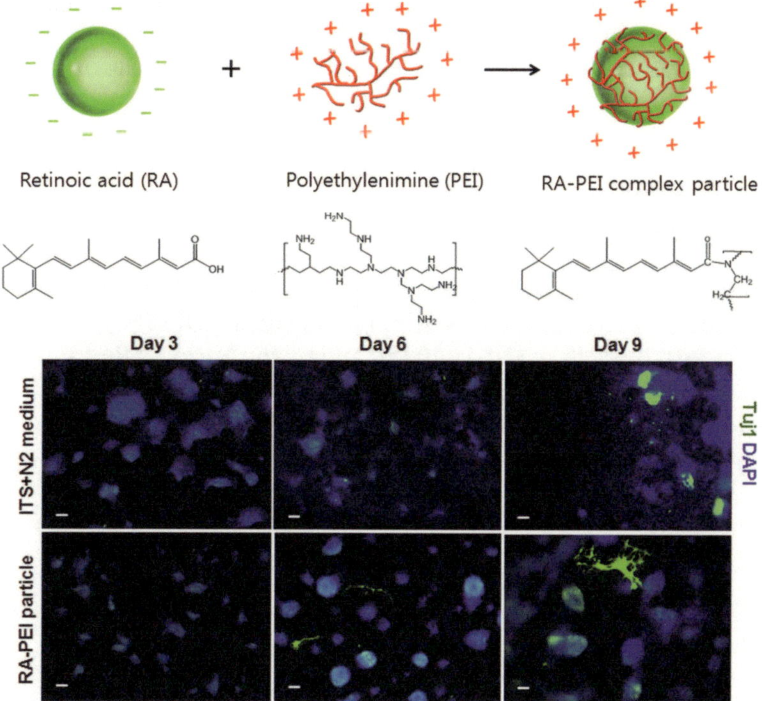

Figure 10.
Applications of nanoparticle for neuronal differentiation: Polyethyleminine (PEI). This study described the synthesis of functional RA-PEI complex nanoparticles with controlled release properties and their effectiveness in inducing neuronal differentiation of embryonic stem (ES) cells, suggesting their potential as a powerful tool for directing murine ES cell fate [75].

6. Summary and outlook

In spite of several long-term efforts to employ biomaterials to improve the physiological relevance of stem cell-derived spinal motor neurons *in vitro*, the resulting cells are still far from representing accurate reflections of their native counterparts in many physiological respects *in vivo*. We believe the core problem lies in the fact that we do not currently have the necessary tools to enable us to recapitulate the dynamic flux of morphogens continuously occurring near the neural tube during the developmental process. One attractive candidate for helping to achieve this goal is micro- and nanotechnology that generates 3D scaffold with high cavity of reservoir for target morphogen loading with a controllable release rate and concentration for longer period of time *in vitro*. By virtue of having established production protocols for those biomaterials with highly tunable porous structure and surface properties, we believe such materials have great potential to function as a morphogen-releasing source that facilitates the establishment of *in vitro* environments corresponding more closely with those of the notochord and paraxial mesoderm.

In conclusion, the use of biocompatible materials has great promise to address a current roadblock in iPSC-neuron research, namely, the accurate recapitulation of native spinal neuron development in culture. Conversion into a 3D culture environment that incorporates materials of similar mechanical and physical properties to those of native extracellular matrices holds great potential to improve current neurodevelopment modeling. More importantly, future efforts to recapitulate the unique morphogen supply schemes present at different stages of spinal cord development in human embryos would help overcome one of the most challenging issues in producing reliable neural tissue models from iPSC-derived spinal neurons.

Acknowledgments

This work was supported by a grant of the Korea Health Technology R&D Project through the Korea Health Industry Development Institute (KHIDI), funded by the Ministry of Health & Welfare (HI19C1095), and by the National Research Foundation of Korea (NRF) grant funded by the Ministry of Science and ICT (RS-2023-00209822), Republic of Korea.

Author details

Juyoung Seong[1], Changho Chun[2], Alec S.T. Smith[2], Jinmyoung Joo[1]*
and David L. Mack[2]*

1 Ulsan National Institute of Science and Technology (UNIST), South Korea

2 University of Washington, Seattle, USA

*Address all correspondence to: dmack21@uw.edu and jjoo@unist.ac.kr

References

[1] Taylor JP, Brown RH Jr, Cleveland DW. Decoding ALS: From genes to mechanism. Nature. 2016;**539**(7628):197-206

[2] Al-Chalabi A, Hardiman O. The epidemiology of ALS: A conspiracy of genes, environment and time. Nature Reviews Neurology. 2013;**9**(11):617-628

[3] Cudkowicz M, McKenna-Yasek D, Sapp P, Chin W, Geller B, Hayden D, et al. Epidemiology of mutations in superoxide dismutase in amyotrophic lateal sclerosis. Annals of Neurology: Official Journal of the American Neurological Association and the Child Neurology Society. 1997;**41**(2):210-221

[4] Poppe L, Rué L, Robberecht W, Van Den Bosch L. Translating biological findings into new treatment strategies for amyotrophic lateral sclerosis (ALS). Experimental Neurology. 2014;**262**:138-151

[5] Kim G, Gautier O, Tassoni-Tsuchida E, Ma XR, Gitler AD. ALS genetics: Gains, losses, and implications for future therapies. Neuron. 2020;**108**(5):822-842

[6] Mercuri E, Sumner CJ, Muntoni F, Darras BT, Finkel RS. Spinal muscular atrophy. Nature Reviews Disease Primers. 2022;**8**(1):52

[7] Pearn J. Incidence, prevalence, and gene frequency studies of chronic childhood spinal muscular atrophy. Journal of Medical Genetics. 1978;**15**(6):409-413

[8] Schnaar R, Schaffner AE. Separation of cell types from embryonic chicken and rat spinal cord: Characterization of motoneuron-enriched fractions. Journal of Neuroscience. 1981;**1**(2):204-217

[9] Kuhn D, Udell W. The development of argument skills. Child Development. 2003;**74**(5):1245-1260

[10] Thorburne SK, Juurlink BH. Low glutathione and high iron govern the susceptibility of oligodendroglial precursors to oxidative stress. Journal of Neurochemistry. 1996;**67**(3):1014-1022

[11] Henderson V, Kuncoro A, Turner M. Industrial development in cities. Journal of Political Economy. 1995;**103**(5):1067-1090

[12] Berg DK, Fischbach GD. Enrichment of spinal cord cell cultures with motoneurons. The Journal of Cell Biology. 1978;**77**(1):83-98

[13] Camu W, Henderson CE. Rapid purification of embryonic rat moteneurons: And in vitro model for studying MND/ALS pathogenesis. Journal of the Neurological Sciences. 1994;**124**:73-74

[14] Camu W, Henderson CE. Purification of embryonic rat motoneurons by panning on a monoclonal antibody to the low-affinity NGF receptor. Journal of Neuroscience Methods. 1992;**44**(1):59-70

[15] Slater CR. The structure of human neuromuscular junctions: Some unanswered molecular questions. International Journal of Molecular Sciences. 2017;**18**(10):2183

[16] Petrov D, Mansfield C, Moussy A, Hermine O. ALS clinical trials review: 20 years of failure. Are we any closer to registering a new treatment? Frontiers in Aging Neuroscience. 2017;**9**:68

[17] Bucchia M, Merwin SJ, Re DB, Kariya S. Limitations and challenges in modeling diseases involving spinal motor

neuron degeneration in vitro. Frontiers in Cellular Neuroscience. 2018;**12**:61

[18] Teschke K, Harris MA, Reynolds CC, Winters M, Babul S, Chipman M, et al. Route infrastructure and the risk of injuries to bicyclists: A case-crossover study. American Journal of Public Health. 2012;**102**(12):2336-2343

[19] Yadav A, Matson KJ, Li L, Hua I, Petrescu J, Kang K, et al. A cellular taxonomy of the adult human spinal cord. Neuron. 2023;**111**(3):328-344 e7

[20] Liu Q, Spusta SC, Mi R, Lassiter RN, Stark MR, Höke A, et al. Human neural crest stem cells derived from human ESCs and induced pluripotent stem cells: Induction, maintenance, and differentiation into functional Schwann cells. Stem Cells Translational Medicine. 2012;**1**(4):266-278

[21] Lin C-Y, Yoshida M, Li L-T, Ikenaka A, Oshima S, Nakagawa K, et al. iPSC-derived functional human neuromuscular junctions model the pathophysiology of neuromuscular diseases. JCI Insight. 2019;**4**(18):1-14. Available from: https://insight.jci.org/articles/view/124299

[22] Lundin A. Human IPSC Derived Neural Cells as Models of Brain Development and as Tools in Pharmaceutical Drug Discovery. Karolinska Institutet (Sweden); 2019. Available from: https://www.proquest.com/docview/2564455343?pq-origsite=gscholar&fromopenview=true

[23] Lanjewar SN, Sloan SA. Growing glia: Cultivating human stem cell models of gliogenesis in health and disease. Frontiers in Cell and Developmental Biology. 2021;**9**:592

[24] Tams D. Use of Enabling Technologies in Combination with Human Pluripotent Stem Cells to Study Neural Differentiation and Neurite Outgrowth. Durham University; 2014. Available from: http://etheses.dur.ac.uk/10528/

[25] Jensen MB, Yan H, Krishnaney-Davison R, Al Sawaf A, Zhang S-C. Survival and differentiation of transplanted neural stem cells derived from human induced pluripotent stem cells in a rat stroke model. Journal of Stroke and Cerebrovascular Diseases. 2013;**22**(4):304-308

[26] Nolte C, De Kumar B, Krumlauf R. Hox genes: Downstream "effectors" of retinoic acid signaling in vertebrate embryogenesis. Genesis. 2019;**57**(7-8):e23306

[27] Paschaki M, Lin S-C, Wong RLY, Finnell RH, Dollé P, Niederreither K. Retinoic acid-dependent signaling pathways and lineage events in the developing mouse spinal cord. PLoS One. 2012;**7**(3):e32447

[28] Marshall H, Studer M, Pöpperl H, Aparicio S, Kuroiwa A, Brenner S, et al. A conserved retinoic acid response element required for early expression of the homeobox gene Hoxb-1. Nature. 1994;**370**(6490):567-571

[29] Maden M, Holder N. Retinoic acid and development of the central nervous system. BioEssays. 1992;**14**(7):431-438

[30] Sances S, Bruijn LI, Chandran S, Eggan K, Ho R, Klim JR, et al. Modeling ALS with motor neurons derived from human induced pluripotent stem cells. Nature Neuroscience. 2016;**19**(4):542-553

[31] Kelleher FC, O'Sullivan H, Smyth E, McDermott R, Viterbo A. Fibroblast growth factor receptors, developmental corruption and malignant disease. Carcinogenesis. 2013;**34**(10):2198-2205

[32] Yu Y, Bai F, Liu Y, Yang Y, Yuan Q, Zou D, et al. Fibroblast growth factor (FGF21) protects mouse liver against D-galactose-induced oxidative stress and apoptosis via activating Nrf2 and PI3K/Akt pathways. Molecular and Cellular Biochemistry. 2015;**403**:287-299

[33] Cheng Y, Zhang J, Guo W, Li F, Sun W, Chen J, et al. Up-regulation of Nrf2 is involved in FGF21-mediated fenofibrate protection against type 1 diabetic nephropathy. Free Radical Biology and Medicine. 2016;**93**:94-109

[34] Lu Y, Li R, Zhu J, Wu Y, Li D, Dong L, et al. Fibroblast growth factor 21 facilitates peripheral nerve regeneration through suppressing oxidative damage and autophagic cell death. Journal of Cellular and Molecular Medicine. 2019;**23**(1):497-511

[35] Du Z-W, Chen H, Liu H, Lu J, Qian K, Huang C-L, et al. Generation and expansion of highly pure motor neuron progenitors from human pluripotent stem cells. Nature Communications. 2015;**6**(1):6626

[36] Davis-Dusenbery BN, Williams LA, Klim JR, Eggan K. How to make spinal motor neurons. Development. 2014;**141**(3):491-501

[37] Petros TJ, Tyson JA, Anderson SA. Pluripotent stem cells for the study of CNS development. Frontiers in Molecular Neuroscience. 2011;**4**:30

[38] El-Sherbiny I, Yacoub M. Hydrogel scaffolds for tissue engineering: Progress and challenges. Global Cardiology Science and Practice. 2013;**38**:1-27. Available from: https://www.qscience.com/content/journals/10.5339/gcsp.2013.38

[39] Lukin I, Erezuma I, Maeso L, Zarate J, Desimone MF, Al-Tel TH, et al. Progress in gelatin as biomaterial for tissue engineering. Pharmaceutics. 2022;**14**(6):1177

[40] Singh A, Elisseeff J. Biomaterials for stem cell differentiation. Journal of Materials Chemistry. 2010;**20**(40):8832-8847

[41] Larsen MT, Kuhlmann M, Hvam ML, Howard KA. Albumin-based drug delivery: Harnessing nature to cure disease. Molecular and Cellular Therapies. 2016;**4**(1):1-12

[42] Hsu C-C, Serio A, Amdursky N, Besnard C, Stevens MM. Fabrication of hemin-doped serum albumin-based fibrous scaffolds for neural tissue engineering applications. ACS Applied Materials & Interfaces. 2018;**10**(6):5305-5317

[43] Amiryaghoubi N, Fathi M, Barzegari A, Barar J, Omidian H, Omidi Y. Recent advances in polymeric scaffolds containing carbon nanotube and graphene oxide for cartilage and bone regeneration. Materials Today Communications. 2021;**26**:102097

[44] Roth JG, Huang MS, Li TL, Feig VR, Jiang Y, Cui B, et al. Advancing models of neural development with biomaterials. Nature Reviews Neuroscience. 2021;**22**(10):593-615

[45] Sthanam LK, Saxena N, Mistari VK, Roy T, Jadhav SR, Sen S. Initial priming on soft substrates enhances subsequent topography-induced neuronal differentiation in ESCs but not in MSCs. ACS Biomaterials Science & Engineering. 2018;**5**(1):180-192

[46] Park SY, Choi DS, Jin HJ, Park J, Byun K-E, Lee K-B, et al. Polarization-controlled differentiation of human neural stem cells using synergistic cues from the patterns of carbon

nanotube monolayer coating. ACS Nano. 2011;**5**(6):4704-4711

[47] Baranes K, Shevach M, Shefi O, Dvir T. Gold nanoparticle-decorated scaffolds promote neuronal differentiation and maturation. Nano Letters. 2016;**16**(5):2916-2920

[48] Patel BB, McNamara MC, Pesquera-Colom LS, Kozik EM, Okuzonu J, Hashemi NN, et al. Recovery of encapsulated adult neural progenitor cells from microfluidic-spun hydrogel fibers enhances proliferation and neuronal differentiation. ACS Omega. 2020;**5**(14):7910-7918

[49] Worthington KS, Green BJ, Rethwisch M, Wiley LA, Tucker BA, Guymon CA, et al. Neuronal differentiation of induced pluripotent stem cells on surfactant templated chitosan hydrogels. Biomacromolecules. 2016;**17**(5):1684-1695

[50] Sun X, Zhang C, Xu J, Zhai H, Liu S, Xu Y, et al. Neurotrophin-3-loaded multichannel nanofibrous scaffolds promoted anti-inflammation, neuronal differentiation, and functional recovery after spinal cord injury. ACS Biomaterials Science & Engineering. 2020;**6**(2):1228-1238

[51] Solanki A, Shah S, Yin PT, Lee K-B. Nanotopography-mediated reverse uptake for siRNA delivery into neural stem cells to enhance neuronal differentiation. Scientific Reports. 2013;**3**(1):1553

[52] Lyon JG, Karumbaiah L, Bellamkonda RV. Neural tissue engineering. In: He B, editor. Neural Engineering. Cham: Springer; 2020. DOI: 10.1007/978-3-030-43395-6_22

[53] Chun J, Bhak G, Lee S-G, Lee J-H, Lee D, Char K, et al. κ-Casein-based hierarchical suprastructures and their use for selective temporal and spatial control over neuronal differentiation. Biomacromolecules. 2012;**13**(9):2731-2738

[54] Kang S, Chen X, Gong S, Yu P, Yau S, Su Z, et al. Characteristic analyses of a neural differentiation model from iPSC-derived neuron according to morphology, physiology, and global gene expression pattern. Scientific Reports. 2017;**7**(1):12233

[55] Urrutia-Cabrera D, Hsiang-Chi Liou R, Lin J, Shi Y, Liu K, Hung SS, et al. Combinatorial approach of binary colloidal crystals and CRISPR activation to improve induced pluripotent stem cell differentiation into neurons. ACS Applied Materials & Interfaces. 2022;**14**(7):8669-8679

[56] Wetzel R, Shivaprasad S, Williams AD. Plasticity of amyloid fibrils. Biochemistry. 2007;**46**(1):1-10

[57] Bhak G, Lee S, Park JW, Cho S, Paik SR. Amyloid hydrogel derived from curly protein fibrils of α-synuclein. Biomaterials. 2010;**31**(23):5986-5995

[58] Xu Y, Chen C, Hellwarth PB, Bao X. Biomaterials for stem cell engineering and biomanufacturing. Bioactive Materials. 2019;**4**:366-379

[59] Causa F, Netti PA, Ambrosio L. A multi-functional scaffold for tissue regeneration: The need to engineer a tissue analogue. Biomaterials. 2007;**28**(34):5093-5099

[60] Willerth SM, Arendas KJ, Gottlieb DI, Sakiyama-Elbert SE. Optimization of fibrin scaffolds for differentiation of murine embryonic stem cells into neural lineage cells. Biomaterials. 2006;**27**(36):5990-6003

[61] Engler AJ, Sen S, Sweeney HL, Discher DE. Matrix elasticity directs stem cell lineage specification. Cell. 2006;**126**(4):677-689

[62] Martino S, D'Angelo F, Armentano I, Kenny JM, Orlacchio A. Stem cell-biomaterial interactions for regenerative medicine. Biotechnology Advances. 2012;**30**(1):338-351

[63] Bianco A, Del Gaudio C, Baiguera S, Armentano I, Bertarelli C, Dottori M, et al. Microstructure and cytocompatibility of electrospun nanocomposites based on poly (ε-caprolactone) and carbon nanostructures. The International Journal of Artificial Organs. 2010;**33**(5):271-282

[64] Baker SC, Rohman G, Southgate J, Cameron NR. The relationship between the mechanical properties and cell behaviour on PLGA and PCL scaffolds for bladder tissue engineering. Biomaterials. 2009;**30**(7):1321-1328

[65] Hong Z, Zhang P, He C, Qiu X, Liu A, Chen L, et al. Nano-composite of poly (L-lactide) and surface grafted hydroxyapatite: Mechanical properties and biocompatibility. Biomaterials. 2005;**26**(32):6296-6304

[66] Sun S, Titushkin I, Cho M. Regulation of mesenchymal stem cell adhesion and orientation in 3D collagen scaffold by electrical stimulus. Bioelectrochemistry. 2006;**69**(2):133-141

[67] Wang E, Zhao M, Forrester JV, McCaig CD. Bi-directional migration of lens epithelial cells in a physiological electrical field. Experimental Eye Research. 2003;**76**(1):29-37

[68] Choi J-W, Seo M, Kim K, Kim A-R, Lee H, Kim H-S, et al. Aptamer nanoconstructs crossing human blood–brain barrier discovered via microphysiological system-based SELEX technology. ACS Nano. 2023;**17**:8153-8166

[69] Maia J, Santos T, Aday S, Agasse F, Cortes L, Malva JO, et al. Controlling the neuronal differentiation of stem cells by the intracellular delivery of retinoic acid-loaded nanoparticles. ACS Nano. 2011;**5**(1):97-106

[70] Park J, Hong K, Carter P, Asgari H, Guo L, Keller G, et al. Development of anti-p185HER2 immunoliposomes for cancer therapy. Proceedings of the National Academy of Sciences. 1995;**92**(5):1327-1331

[71] Rip J, Chen L, Hartman R, van den Heuvel A, Reijerkerk A, van Kregten J, et al. Glutathione PEGylated liposomes: Pharmacokinetics and delivery of cargo across the blood–brain barrier in rats. Journal of Drug Targeting. 2014;**22**(5):460-467

[72] Ma W, Shao X, Zhao D, Li Q, Liu M, Zhou T, et al. Self-assembled tetrahedral DNA nanostructures promote neural stem cell proliferation and neuronal differentiation. ACS Applied Materials & Interfaces. 2018;**10**(9):7892-7900

[73] Cho Y-W, Jee S, Suhito IR, Lee J-H, Park CG, Choi KM, et al. Single metal-organic framework–embedded nanopit arrays: A new way to control neural stem cell differentiation. Science Advances. 2022;**8**(16):eabj7736

[74] Park S-J, Kim S, Kim S-Y, Jeon NL, Song JM, Won C, et al. Highly efficient and rapid neural differentiation of mouse embryonic stem cells based on retinoic acid encapsulated porous nanoparticle. ACS Applied Materials & Interfaces. 2017;**9**(40):34634-34640

[75] Ku B, Kim J-E, Chung BH, Chung BG. Retinoic acid-polyethyleneimine complex nanoparticles for embryonic stem cell-derived neuronal differentiation. Langmuir. 2013;**29**(31):9857-9862

[76] Santos T, Ferreira R, Maia J, Agasse F, Xapelli S, Cortes L, et al. Polymeric nanoparticles to control the differentiation of neural stem cells in the subventricular zone of the brain. ACS Nano. 2012;**6**(12):10463-10474

Chapter 4

The Endocannabinoid System as a Potential Therapeutic Target for Amyotrophic Lateral Sclerosis

Kamila Saramak and Natalia Szejko

Abstract

Amyotrophic lateral sclerosis (ALS) is a fatal neurodegenerative disease characterized by a selective loss of motor neurons from the spinal cord, brainstem and motor cortex. With a prevalence of about 5.5–9.9 per 100,000 persons, ALS is the most common form of motor neuron disease (MND). Although the mechanisms underlying the pathophysiology of this condition are not yet fully understood, it is believed that excitotoxicity, inflammation and oxidative stress play an important role in selective motor neuron death. Despite intensive research, up to this point no cure for ALS has been identified. There is increasing evidence that cannabinoids, due to their anti-glutamatergic and anti-inflammatory actions, may show neuroprotective effects in ALS patients and slow the progression of the disease. Furthermore, cannabis-based medicine may be useful in managing symptoms like pain, spasticity or weight loss. The aim of this chapter is to summarize the current state of research regarding the efficacy and safety of medical cannabis in the treatment of ALS.

Keywords: motor neuron disease, amyotrophic lateral sclerosis, neuroprotection, endocannabinoids, cannabis

1. Introduction

Amyotrophic lateral sclerosis (ALS) is a multisystem neurodegenerative disease leading to the progressive degradation of both upper (UMN) and lower motor neurons (LMN). With its prevalence of about 5.5–9.9 per 100,000 persons, ALS is the most common form of motor neuron disease (MND) [1]. The condition affects primarily the pyramidal motor system, including the motor cortex, cranial nerve motor nuclei and spinal cord motor neurons. The mean age of onset of sporadic ALS is about 60 years with a higher incidence among males [2]. The majority of ALS patients present with limb onset of the disease, resulting in focal muscle weakness and atrophy. Over time, due to the damage of the upper motor neurons, spasticity develops. On the other hand, patients with bulbar onset of ALS initially report dysarthria and dysphagia. The limb symptoms may occur almost simultaneously with bulbar symptoms, and in most cases develop within 1–2 years [3]. Subsequently, the disease involves various body regions, in particular respiratory muscles, causing death within 2–3 years

IntechOpen

for bulbar onset cases and 3–5 years for limb onset cases [4]. The neurodegeneration progresses in the neighboring cortical regions, including the prefrontal cortex, ventral and medial frontal cortical areas, and eventually involves portions of the parietal and temporal lobes and the deep gray structures. This results in non-motor symptoms of the disease such as impairment of executive functions, behavioral changes and language disorders in up to 50% of cases [5]. The cognitive decline in 10–15% of ALS patients is consistent with the diagnosis of frontotemporal dementia (FTD) [6]. To date, the only therapy widely approved for ALS is an anti-glutamate agent riluzole. It has been proven that riluzole slows the progression of ALS, extends survival and delays the time to tracheostomy. The benefit is, however, very limited and riluzole can extend the average survival time by only 3 months [7, 8]. Another drug, edaravone, was first approved in Japan, followed by South Korea, U.S., Canada, Switzerland, and China. Edaravone is a free radical scavenger that can reduce oxidative stress. Its beneficial clinical effects have been initially proven in Japan [9]. The subsequent study in the USA has showed that an intravenous treatment with edaravone prolonged the survival for 6 months [10]. These findings, however, have not been confirmed in the European cohorts [11, 12]. The third drug, AMX0035 has been approved for the treatment of ALS in the USA and Canada. AMX0035 is a combination of two compounds – tauroursodeoxycholic acid (TUDCA) and sodium phenylbutyrate (PB). It is thought to increase the threshold for cell death by blocking key cell death pathways and reducing the stress on the endoplasmic reticulum (ER) simultaneously [13]. The first randomized, placebo-controlled, phase 2 trial of AMX0035 in ALS (CENTAUR) has shown both functional and survival benefits in ALS patients [14]. Moreover, there are many experimental therapies in development, most of them showing anti-inflammatory and anti- excitotoxic mechanisms of action [15].

2. Possible role of the endocannabinoid system in the motor neuron disease

In recent decades, the endocannabinoid system has been gaining increasing attention as a potential therapeutic target in a number of neurological disorders [16, 17]. Thus far, two cannabinoid receptors (CB) have been identified: the CB receptor type 1 (CB1) and CB receptor type 2 (CB2), both belonging to the G protein-coupled receptors (GPCRs) family. The CB1 is expressed primarily in the central nervous system (CNS), especially in the neocortex, hippocampus, basal ganglia, cerebellum, and brainstem [18]. Apart from the CNS, CB1 has also been identified in numerous peripheral tissues and cell types [19]. On the other hand, the CB2 receptor is abundantly present in the immune system and in smaller quantities in the CNS, especially in human microglia [20].

Although a wide range of dysfunctional cellular processes related to neurodegeneration in ALS has been described, the exact mechanisms underlying its pathogenesis remain largely unknown. Mutations in more than 30 different genes associated with diverse molecular functions has been linked to ALS, which explains approximately 20% cases of the disease [21]. A process of excessive activation of glutamate receptors, resulting in neuronal dysfunction and death called "excitotoxicity" is believed to play an important role in the pathogenesis of many neurological disorders, including ALS [22]. Elevated extracellular glutamate levels activate postsynaptic glutamate receptors, causing an increased influx of calcium into the postsynaptic neurons. Subsequently, excessive postsynaptic calcium activates neurotoxic cascades, resulting in neuronal death. The activation of N-methyl-D-aspartate (NMDA) receptors may lead to cellular death more rapidly than the activation of α-amino-3-hydroxy-5-methyl-4-isoxazolepropionic (AMPA) and kainite receptors [23]. Studies *in vitro* and *in vivo* have shown that activation of cannabinoid receptors may inhibit neuronal hyperexcitability associated with activation of both NMDA and non-NMDA subtypes of glutamate receptors [24–27]. Similarly, the potent anti-inflammatory properties of cannabinoids may be used to reduce chronic neuroinflammation and thus prevent motor neuron toxicity. Both CB1 and CB2 receptors were found to modulate release of endogenous interleukin-1 receptor antagonist (IL-1ra) from primary cultured glial cells, exerting neuroprotective effects [28]. Moreover, recent studies proved the anti-oxidative properties of cannabis, in particular inhibition of oxidative and nitrosative stress as well as reduced production of reactive oxygen species (ROS) [29]. CBD has been also found to regulate mitochondrial calcium concentrations as well as mitochondria-mediated intrinsic apoptosis [30, 31]. Additionally, CBD treatment may exert beneficial effects on skeletal muscle by reducing inflammation and improving muscle recovery [32].

3. Neuroprotective effects of cannabinoids in animal models of ALS

The most commonly used animal model to explore ALS is the SOD (G93A) transgenic mouse. The mouse is genetically engineered to express a mutation in the superoxide dismutase-1 gene (SOD1-G93A) and thus shows a phenotype similar to ALS in humans [33]. Raman et al. have demonstrated, that treatment with delta-9-tetrahydrocannabinol (Δ^9-THC) in ALS SOD1 mice improved motor deficits and increased survival by 5%, most probably due to its anti glutamatergic and anti-oxidant mechanisms of action [34]. Weydt et al. have shown, that cannabinol (CBN), a nonpsychotropic cannabinoid, delayed symptom onset in SOD1 transgenic mice without improving the survival [35]. In the subsequent study, Bilsland et al. have investigated the postsymptomatic treatment with an exogenous synthetic cannabinoid as well as genetic augmentation of endocannabinoids. The group has proven, that a potent CB1 and CB2 receptor agonist, WIN 55, 212-2, delayed the disease progression without affecting survival [36]. On the contrary, Shoemaker et al. have demonstrated, that a selective CB2 agonist, AM-1241, extended the lifespan of SOD1 mice by 4%, while WIN 55, 212-2 extended it by even 11% [37]. Zhao et al. have strengthened the evidence for AM-1241, showing its beneficial effect on disease progression [38]. Consequently, Moreno et al. evaluated the efficacy of nabiximols (trade name Sativex®) in SOD1 mice for the first time. Sativex® is a combination of 2.5 mg of CBD and 2.7 mg of Δ9-THC in the form of an oromucosal spray. In this study, Sativex® proved to be effective both in slowing the disease progression and improving survival [39]. Pasquarelli et al. have examined the neuroprotective and anti-inflammatory properties of 2-arachidonoylglycerol (2-AG). 2-AG is an endogenous CB1 and CB2 receptor agonist, which is present at relatively high levels in the central nervous system and is degraded by monoacylglycerol lipase (MAGL). In this study, the MAGL inhibitor KML29 was applied in order to increase the concentration of the 2-AG in the CNS of the SOD1 transgenic mice. This led to a reduction of proinflammatory cytokines and an increase in brain-derived neurotrophic factor (BDNF) expression levels in the spinal cord, the major site of neurodegeneration in ALS. Moreover, the oral KML29 treatment delayed the disease onset and extended life span in SOD1 mice up to 24 days [40]. Espejo- Porras et al. used another animal

Reference	Model	Substance	Outcome
Raman et al. [34]	SOD1 mice	Δ^9-THC	Δ^9-THC delayed disease progression in SOD1 mice and expanded their lifespan by 5%.
Weydt et al. [35]	SOD1 mice	cannabinol	Cannabinol delayed disease onset in SOD1 mice.
Bilsland et al. [36]	SOD1mice	WIN 55, 212-2 CB1 and Faah ablation	Delayed disease progression in SOD1 mice. Expanded lifespan in SOD1 mice by 13%.
Shoemaker et al. [37]	SOD1 mice	AM-1241 WIN-55,212-2	AM-1241 extended lifespan of SOD1 mice by 4% WIN-55,212-2 extended lifespan of SOD1 mice by 11%
Zhao et al. [38]	SOD1 mice	AM-1241	Delayed disease progression in SOD1 mice.
Moreno et al. [39]	SOD1 mice	combination of cannabidiol and Δ^9-THC (Sativex®)	Delayed disease progression in SOD1 mice and improved survival.
Pasquarelli et al. [40]	SOD1 mice	2-AG	Delayed disease progression in SOD1 mice and improved survival.
Espejo- Porras et al. [41]	TDP-43 (A315T) mice	WIN55,212-2 HU-308	Delayed disease progression in TDP-43 mice.
Rodriguez-Cueto [42]	SOD1 mice	VCE-003.2	Improved survival of spinal motor neurons. Delayed disease progression in SOD-1 mice.

SOD 1, superoxide dismutase-1; Δ9-THC, Δ9-tetrahydrocannabinol; FAAH, fatty acid amide hydrolase; CB1, Cannabinoid receptor type 1; 2-AG, 2-arachidonoylglycerol.

Table 1.
Summary of studies exploring the endocannabinoid system in animal models of ALS. Studies are presented in chronological order.

model, TDP-43 transgenic mice. The mis-metabolism of the RNA/DNA-binding protein TDP-43 (ALS-TDP), in particular, the presence of cytosolic aggregates of the protein is found in the spinal cords of more than 95% of ALS patients. Both the non-selective agonist WIN55,212-2 alone as well as in combination with the selective CB2 agonist HU-308 were shown to delay disease progression in TDP-43 mice [41]. Rodriguez-Cueto explored the anti-inflammatory, anti-oxidative and neuroprotective properties of VCE-003.2. VCE-003.2 is a novel derivative of the non-psychotrophic phytocannabinoid cannabigerol (CBG), which activates the peroxisome proliferator-activated receptor-γ (PPARγ). The treatment with VCE-003.2 was associated with a strong preservation of spinal motor neurons which may be attributed to normalizing the activation and cell function of the astrocytes [42]. An overview of studies investigating the endocannabinoid system in animal models of ALS is shown in **Table 1**.

4. Clinical research with cannabis-based medicine in ALS

In 2004 Amtmann et al. conducted the first survey on marijuana use among 131 patients with ALS. In this group of patients, 13 males reported using cannabis in the previous 12 months. Cannabis smokers reported reduction of depression, appetite loss, pain, spasticity, drooling and weakness [43]. To date, only a very limited number of studies regarding the potential use of CBM in ALS has been conducted. A small pilot study conducted by Gelinas et al. in a group of 20 ALS patients found THC to be effective against muscle cramps, fasciculations, insomnia and lack of appetite [44]. Subsequently, Weber et al. investigated the efficacy of oral THC in the treatment of ALS-related cramps in a group of 27 patients. The participants were randomly assigned to receive 5 mg THC twice daily followed by placebo or *vice versa* for 2 weeks. The intensity of cramps was assessed using the visual analogue scale (VAS). Unfortunately, no statistically significant improvement of cramp intensity, number of cramps, or fasciculation intensity was observed. No serious adverse events were noted, one of the participants complained about dizziness [45]. Joerger et al. examined the pharmacokinetics (PK) and tolerability of oral THC in ALS patients. The group showed, that adverse events (drowsiness, euphoria, orthostasis, sleepiness, vertigo and weakness) occurred more frequently in patients receiving 10 mg compared to 5 mg THC. No serious adverse events were reported. A marked interindividual variability regarding the absorption and elimination of THC was also observed [46]. Meyer et al. explored the efficacy of nabiximols in the treatment of ALS – related spasticity in a retrospective, mono-centric cohort study with 32 patients. The participants were treated with an oromucosal spray, the mean dose was 5.5 actuations per day. Spasticity was rated using the Numering Rating Scale (NRS) and the patient's experience was evaluated with the net promoter score (NPS) and treatment satisfaction questionnaire (TSMQ-9). Moderate to severe spasticity was associated with an

Reference	Number of patients	Substance	Results	Safety
Gelinas et al. [44]	20	oral Δ 9-THC	Improvement of effective against muscle cramps, fasciculations, insomnia and lack of appetite.	No data.
Weber et al. [45]	22	oral Δ 9-THC	No significant improvement of cramp intensity, number of cramps, or fasciculation intensity.	No study-related SAEs. AEs: dizziness.
Joerger et al. [46]	9	oral Δ 9-THC	AEs more frequent in patients receiving 10 mg compared to 5 mg THC. A marked interindividual variability regarding the absorption and elimination of THC.	No study-related SAEs. AEs: drowsiness, euphoria, orthostasis, sleepiness, vertigo, and weakness
Meyer et al. [47]	32	nabiximols (Sativex®)	Higher efficacy in subgroups of ALS patients with moderate to severe spasticity. High treatment satisfaction (TSQM-9).	Not data.
Riva et al. [48]	59	nabiximols (Sativex®)	Significant reduction of ALS-related spasticity	No SAEs. AEs: asthenia, somnolence, vertigo, and nausea.

Δ9-THC, Δ9-tetrahydrocannabinol; AEs, adverse events; SAEs, Serious Adverse Events.

Table 2.
Summary of clinical studies investigating the efficacy and safety of the cannabis – Based medicine in ALS patients. Studies are presented in chronological order.

elevated number of daily THC:CBD actuations and stronger recommendation rate (NPS) [47]. A larger, multicentre, double-blind, randomized, placebo-controlled study (CANALS) was conducted by Riva et al. The group investigated the efficacy of nabiximols (trade name Sativex®) in the treatment of ALS-related spasticity in a group of 59 patients (29 in the nabiximols group and 30 in the placebo group). The participants self-titrated the oromucosal spray during the first 2 weeks of treatment, receiving up to 12 puffs per day, then maintained the dose for 4 weeks. After 6 weeks of treatment a statistically significant reduction of spasticity evaluated with the Modified Asworth Scale (MAS) was observed in the nabiximols group. No serious adverse events occurred in either group. The most common adverse effects in the nabiximols group were asthenia, somnolence, vertigo, and nausea [48]. Only recently, the EMERALD trial, a randomized, double-blind, placebo-controlled study was initiated to investigate the efficacy of cannabis-based medicine (CBME) on slowing down the progression of ALS. The investigational product contains 25 mg of CBD and less than 2 mg of THC (approximately 10%) formulated as a capsule. A total number of 30 patients with probable or definite ALS diagnosis based on the El Escorial criteria, with the symptom duration of <2 years, has been included in the study. The primary objective of the study is to evaluate the efficacy of CMBE on the disease progression measured with ALS Functional Rating Scale-Revised and forced vital capacity (FVC) score after 6 months of treatment [49].

An overview of clinical studies investigating the efficacy and safety of the cannabis – based medicine in ALS patients is shown in **Table 2**.

5. Safety profile of cannabis-based medicine in patients with ALS

Thus far, very little is known about the safety and tolerability of CBM in patients with ALS. The only study focusing specifically on the tolerability of oral THC showed, that adverse events (drowsiness, euphoria, orthostasis, sleepiness, vertigo, and weakness) were more frequent in ALS patients receiving 10 mg compared to 5 mg THC [46]. This contrasts with findings in patients with multiple sclerosis and healthy subjects [50], who tolerated single doses even up to 15 mg without significant adverse events [51]. However, the abovementioned study included only 10 participants [46]. The other available preliminary results suggested that the safety profile of CBM in ALS is similar to that in other groups of patients and did not report any serious adverse events [45, 47, 48]. A meta-analysis conducted by Whiting, including diverse populations of patients treated with CBM, showed that the treatment with cannabinoids can be associated with a greater risk of adverse events (AE), including serious adverse events (SAE). The most common short-term AEs encompass dizziness, dry mouth, nausea or vomiting, fatigue, somnolence, euphoria, disorientation, drowsiness, confusion, loss of balance, and hallucinations. Moreover, up to this date no study evaluating the long-term AEs of cannabinoids has been conducted [52].

6. Conclusions

Taking into consideration the above-mentioned reports, there is a valid rationale for the use of cannabis-based medicine in the symptomatic treatment of patients with ALS. The efficacy of cannabis in the management of spasticity, drooling and anorexia has been proven not only in the small RCTs with ALS patients, but also in large RTCs including other groups of patients suffering from similar symptoms in the course of other neurological diseases, most commonly in multiple sclerosis (MS) patients. Moreover, there is increasing evidence that cannabinoid compounds may exert neuroprotective effects and prolong the survival in the animal models of ALS. Therefore, larger RTCs are urgently needed to confirm the therapeutic potential of cannabis in slowing down the disease progression.

Author details

Kamila Saramak[1] and Natalia Szejko[2,3]*

1 Department of Neurology, Hochzirl Hospital, Zirl, Austria

2 Department of Clinical Neurosciences, University of Calgary, Alberta, Canada

3 Department of Bioethics, Medical University of Warsaw, Poland

*Address all correspondence to: natalia.szejlo@gmail.com

References

[1] Mehta P, Raymond J, Punjani R, Han M, Larson T, Kaye W, et al. Prevalence of amyotrophic lateral sclerosis in the United States using established and novel methodologies. Amyotrophic Lateral Sclerosis and Frontotemporal Degeneration. 2017;**2022**:1-9

[2] Feldman EL, Goutman SA, Petri S, Mazzini L, Savelieff MG, Shaw PJ, et al. Amyotrophic lateral sclerosis. The Lancet. 2022;**400**:1363-1380

[3] Grossman M. Amyotrophic lateral sclerosis—A multisystem neurodegenerative disorder. Nature Reviews Neurology. 2019;**15**:5-6

[4] Masrori P, Van Damme P. Amyotrophic lateral sclerosis: A clinical review. European Journal of Neurology. 2020;**27**:1918-1929

[5] Crockford C, Newton J, Lonergan K, Chiwera T, Booth T, Chandran S, et al. ALS-specific cognitive and behavior changes associated with advancing disease stage in ALS. Neurology. 2018;**91**:e1370-e1e80

[6] Burrell JR, Halliday GM, Kril JJ, Ittner LM, Götz J, Kiernan MC, et al. The frontotemporal dementia-motor neuron disease continuum. The Lancet. 2016;**388**:919-931

[7] Lacomblez L, Bensimon G, Leigh PN, Guillet P, Meininger V. Dose-ranging study of riluzole in amyotrophic lateral sclerosis. Amyotrophic lateral sclerosis/Riluzole study group II. Lancet. 1996;**347**:1425-1431

[8] Bensimon G, Lacomblez L, Meininger V, Group ARS. A controlled trial of riluzole in amyotrophic lateral sclerosis. New England Journal of Medicine. 1994;**330**:585-591

[9] Abe K, Aoki M, Tsuji S, Itoyama Y, Sobue G, Togo M, et al. Safety and efficacy of edaravone in well defined patients with amyotrophic lateral sclerosis: A randomised, double-blind, placebo-controlled trial. The Lancet Neurology. 2017;**16**:505-512

[10] Brooks BR, Berry JD, Ciepielewska M, Liu Y, Zambrano GS, Zhang J, et al. Intravenous edaravone treatment in ALS and survival: An exploratory, retrospective, administrative claims analysis. EClinicalMedicine. 2022;**52**:101590

[11] Witzel S, Maier A, Steinbach R, Grosskreutz J, Koch JC, Sarikidi A, et al. Safety and effectiveness of long-term intravenous administration of edaravone for treatment of patients with amyotrophic lateral sclerosis. JAMA Neurology. 2022;**79**:121-130

[12] Lunetta C, Moglia C, Lizio A, Caponnetto C, Dubbioso R, Giannini F, et al. The Italian multicenter experience with edaravone in amyotrophic lateral sclerosis. Journal of Neurology. 2020;**267**:3258-3267

[13] Paganoni S, Macklin EA, Hendrix S, Berry JD, Elliott MA, Maiser S, et al. Trial of sodium phenylbutyrate–taurursodiol for amyotrophic lateral sclerosis. New England Journal of Medicine. 2020;**383**:919-930

[14] Paganoni S, Hendrix S, Dickson SP, Knowlton N, Macklin EA, Berry JD, et al. Long-term survival of participants in the CENTAUR trial of sodium phenylbutyrate-taurursodiol in amyotrophic lateral sclerosis. Muscle & Nerve. 2021;**63**:31-39

[15] Jiang J, Wang Y, Deng M. New developments and opportunities in drugs being trialed for amyotrophic lateral sclerosis from 2020 to 2022. Frontiers in Pharmacology. 2022;**13**:2004025

[16] Saramak K, Szejko N. Endocannabinoid System as a New Therapeutic Avenue for the Treatment of Huntington's Disease. In: From Pathophysiology to Treatment of Huntington's Disease. IntechOpen; 2022

[17] Szejko N, Saramak K, Lombroso A, Müller-Vahl K. Cannabis-based medicine in treatment of patients with Gilles de la Tourette syndrome. Neurologia i neurochirurgia polska. 2022;**56**:28-38

[18] Marsicano G, Kuner R. Anatomical distribution of receptors, ligands and enzymes in the brain and in the spinal cord: Circuitries and neurochemistry. Cannabinoids and the Brain. 2008:161-201

[19] Howlett AC, Blume LC, Dalton GD. CB1 cannabinoid receptors and their associated proteins. Current medicinal Chemistry. 2010;**17**:1382-1393

[20] Klegeris A, Bissonnette CJ, McGeer PL. Reduction of human monocytic cell neurotoxicity and cytokine secretion by ligands of the cannabinoid-type CB2 receptor. British Journal of Pharmacology. 2003;**139**:775-786

[21] Turner MR, Al-Chalabi A, Chio A, Hardiman O, Kiernan MC, Rohrer JD, et al. Genetic screening in sporadic ALS and FTD. Journal of Neurology, Neurosurgery & Psychiatry. 2017;**88**:1042

[22] Van Den Bosch L, Van Damme P, Bogaert E, Robberecht W. The role of excitotoxicity in the pathogenesis of amyotrophic lateral sclerosis. Biochimica et Biophysica Acta -Molecular Basis of Disease. 2006;**1762**:1068-1082

[23] Choi DW. Excitotoxic cell death. Journal of Neurobiology. 1992;**23**:1261-1276

[24] Kim SH, Won SJ, Mao XO, Jin K, Greenberg DA. Molecular mechanisms of cannabinoid protection from neuronal excitotoxicity. Molecular Pharmacology. 2006;**69**:691-696

[25] Abood ME, Rizvi G, Sallapudi N, McAllister SD. Activation of the CB1 cannabinoid receptor protects cultured mouse spinal neurons against excitotoxicity. Neuroscience Letters. 2001;**309**:197-201

[26] Marsicano G, Goodenough S, Monory K, Hermann H, Eder M, Cannich A, et al. CB1 cannabinoid receptors and on-demand defense against excitotoxicity. Science. 2003;**302**:84-88

[27] Liu Q, Bhat M, Bowen WD, Cheng J. Signaling pathways from cannabinoid receptor-1 activation to inhibition of N-methyl-D-aspartic acid mediated calcium influx and neurotoxicity in dorsal root ganglion neurons. Journal of Pharmacology and Experimental Therapeutics. 2009;**331**:1062-1070

[28] Molina-Holgado F, Pinteaux E, Moore JD, Molina-Holgado E, Guaza C, Gibson RM, et al. Endogenous interleukin-1 receptor antagonist mediates anti-inflammatory and neuroprotective actions of cannabinoids in neurons and glia. Journal of Neuroscience. 2003;**23**:6470-6474

[29] Velayudhan L, Van Diepen E, Marudkar M, Hands O, Suribhatla S, Prettyman R, et al. Therapeutic potential of cannabinoids in neurodegenerative disorders: A selective review. Current Pharmaceutical Design. 2014;**20**:2218-2230

[30] Ryan D, Drysdale AJ, Lafourcade C, Pertwee RG, Platt B. Cannabidiol targets

mitochondria to regulate intracellular Ca2+ levels. Journal of Neuroscience. 2009;**29**(7):2053-2063

[31] Gross C, Ramirez DA, McGrath S, Gustafson DL. Cannabidiol induces apoptosis and perturbs mitochondrial function in human and canine glioma cells. Frontiers in Pharmacology. 2021;**12**:725136

[32] Schouten M, Dalle S, Koppo K. Molecular mechanisms through which Cannabidiol may affect skeletal muscle metabolism, inflammation, tissue regeneration, and anabolism: A narrative review. Cannabis & Cannabinoid Research. 2022;**7**:745-757

[33] Kim BW, Ryu J, Jeong YE, Kim J, Martin LJ. Human motor neurons with SOD1-G93A mutation generated from CRISPR/Cas9 gene-edited iPSCs develop pathological features of amyotrophic lateral sclerosis. Frontiers in Cellular Neuroscience. 2020;**14**:604171

[34] Raman C, McAllister SD, Rizvi G, Patel SG, Moore DH, Abood ME. Amyotrophic lateral sclerosis: Delayed disease progression in mice by treatment with a cannabinoid. Amyotrophic Lateral Sclerosis Other Motor Neuron Disorders. 2004;**5**:33-39

[35] Weydt P, Hong S, Witting A, Möller T, Stella N, Kliot M. Cannabinol delays symptom onset in SOD1 (G93A) transgenic mice without affecting survival. Amyotrophic Lateral Sclerosis. 2005;**6**:182-184

[36] Bilsland LG, Dick J, Pryce G, Petrosino S, Di Marzo V, Baker D, et al. Increasing cannabinoid levels by pharmacological and genetic manipulation delay disease progression in SOD1 mice. FASEB Journal: Official Publication of the Federation of American Societies for Experimental Biology. 2006;**20**:1003-1005

[37] Shoemaker JL, Seely KA, Reed RL, Crow JP, Prather PL. The CB2 cannabinoid agonist AM-1241 prolongs survival in a transgenic mouse model of amyotrophic lateral sclerosis when initiated at symptom onset. Journal of Neurochemistry. 2007;**101**:87-98

[38] Zhao P, Ignacio S, Beattie EC, Abood ME. Altered presymptomatic AMPA and cannabinoid receptor trafficking in motor neurons of ALS model mice: Implications for excitotoxicity. European Journal of Neuroscience. 2008;**27**:572-579

[39] Moreno-Martet M, Espejo-Porras F, Fernández-Ruiz J, de Lago E. Changes in endocannabinoid receptors and enzymes in the spinal cord of SOD 1G93A transgenic mice and evaluation of a Sativex®-like combination of phytocannabinoids: Interest for future therapies in amyotrophic lateral sclerosis. CNS Neuroscience Therapeutics. 2014;**20**:809-815

[40] Pasquarelli N, Engelskirchen M, Hanselmann J, Endres S, Porazik C, Bayer H, et al. Evaluation of monoacylglycerol lipase as a therapeutic target in a transgenic mouse model of ALS. Neuropharmacology. 2017;**124**:157-169

[41] Espejo-Porras F, García-Toscano L, Rodríguez-Cueto C, Santos-García I, de Lago E, Fernandez-Ruiz J. Targeting glial cannabinoid CB2 receptors to delay the progression of the pathological phenotype in TDP-43 (A315T) transgenic mice, a model of amyotrophic lateral sclerosis. British Journal of Pharmacology. 2019;**176**:1585-1600

[42] Rodríguez-Cueto C, Santos-García I, García-Toscano L, Espejo-Porras F, Bellido M, Fernández-Ruiz J, et al. Neuroprotective effects of the cannabigerol quinone derivative

VCE-003.2 in SOD1G93A transgenic mice, an experimental model of amyotrophic lateral sclerosis. Biochemical Pharmacology. 2018;**157**:217-226

[43] Amtmann D, Weydt P, Johnson KL, Jensen MP, Carter GT. Survey of cannabis use in patients with amyotrophic lateral sclerosis. American Journal of Hospice and Palliative Medicine. 2004;**21**:95-104

[44] Gelinas D, Miller R, Abood M. A pilot study of safety and tolerability of Delta 9-THC (Marinol) treatment for ALS. Amyotrophic Lateral Sclerosis and Other Motor Neuron Disorders. 2002;**3**:23-24

[45] Weber M, Goldman B, Truniger S. Tetrahydrocannabinol (THC) for cramps in amyotrophic lateral sclerosis: A randomised, double-blind crossover trial. Journal of Neurology, Neurosurgery & Psychiatry. 2010;**81**:1135-1140

[46] Joerger M, Wilkins J, Fagagnini S, Baldinger R, Brenneisen R, Schneider U, et al. Single-dose pharmacokinetics and tolerability of oral delta-9-tetrahydrocannabinol in patients with amyotrophic lateral sclerosis. Drug Metabolism Letters. 2012;**6**:102-108

[47] Meyer T, Funke A, Münch C, Kettemann D, Maier A, Walter B, et al. Real world experience of patients with amyotrophic lateral sclerosis (ALS) in the treatment of spasticity using tetrahydrocannabinol: Cannabidiol (THC: CBD). BMC Neurology. 2019;**19**:1-13

[48] Riva N, Mora G, Sorarù G, Lunetta C, Ferraro OE, Falzone Y, et al. Safety and efficacy of nabiximols on spasticity symptoms in patients with motor neuron disease (CANALS): A multicentre, double-blind, randomised, placebo-controlled, phase 2 trial. The Lancet Neurology. 2019;**18**:155-164

[49] Urbi B, Broadley S, Bedlack R, Russo E, Sabet A. Study protocol for a randomised, double-blind, placebo-controlled study evaluating the efficacy of cannabis-based medicine extract in slowing the disease pRogression of amyotrophic lateral sclerosis or motor neurone disease: The EMERALD trial. BMJ Open. 2019;**9**:e029449

[50] Killestein J, Hoogervorst E, Reif M, Kalkers N, Van Loenen A, Staats P, et al. Safety, tolerability, and efficacy of orally administered cannabinoids in MS. Neurology. 2002;**58**:1404-1407

[51] Naef M, Curatolo M, Petersen-Felix S, Arendt-Nielsen L, Zbinden A, Brenneisen R. The analgesic effect of oral delta-9-tetrahydrocannabinol (THC), morphine, and a THC-morphine combination in healthy subjects under experimental pain conditions. Pain. 2003;**105**:79-88

[52] Whiting PF, Wolff RF, Deshpande S, Di Nisio M, Duffy S, Hernandez AV, et al. Cannabinoids for medical use: A systematic review and meta-analysis. Journal of the American Medical Association. 2015;**313**:2456-2473

Chapter 5

Motor Neuron Disease and Delicate Anesthesia Choices – Anesthesia for Motor Neuron Disease Patients

Wendy Wenqiao Yang

Abstract

Motor neuron diseases (MNDs), two major types of which are amyotrophic lateral sclerosis (ALS) and spinal muscular atrophy (SMA), are caused by upper and/or lower motor neuron degeneration and death. They manifest with progressive skeletal muscle atrophy. Most ALS cases are idiopathic, whereas the cause of SMA is genetic. There is no cure for MNDs and anesthetic management is challenging due to patients' respiratory dysfunction, abnormal response to muscle relaxants, and high risk of aspiration. General guidelines for this purpose state that intravenous administration of propofol and remifentanil are preferred. Muscle relaxants should be used sparingly due to their causing ventilatory depression, and depolarizing neuromuscular blockers should be avoided entirely for patients' risk of hyperkalemia. This chapter discusses the etiology of MNDs, their clinical features, disease prognosis, palliative treatments, necessary surgical procedures, and preoperative and postoperative anesthetic management. It covers ALS, SMA, and other less common MNDs.

Keywords: motor neuron disease, muscle atrophy, muscle weakness, general anesthesia, regional anesthesia, muscle relaxants, amyotrophic lateral sclerosis (ALS), spinal muscular atrophy (SMA)

1. Introduction

Motor neuron diseases (MNDs) are a type of neurodegenerative disease caused by upper and/or lower motor neuron axon demyelination and eventual cell demise. Amyotrophic lateral sclerosis (ALS) and spinal muscular atrophy (SMA) are the two major MNDs. While in ALS both upper and lower motor neurons undergo degeneration [1], SMA results from lower motor neuron loss [2]. The cause of ALS, typically in males aged 50–70 years, is unknown, whereas mutations in Survival Motor Neuron-1 (SMN1) gene trigger SMA starting in infancy. Other MNDs that will be discussed include progressive muscular atrophy, primary lateral sclerosis, Kennedy's disease, pseudobulbar palsy, and hereditary spastic paraplegia.

IntechOpen

Based on the Global Burden of Disease, Injuries and Risk Factor (GBD) study, the MND prevalence and attributed deaths in 2019 increased 1.91% and 12.39%, respectively from 1990 [3]. The disease burden of MNDs is increasing; currently, there are an estimated 268,673 MND cases globally [3]. In 2019, MNDs resulted in 1,034,606 disability-adjusted life-years and 39,081 deaths worldwide [3].

The major clinical manifestation of MNDs include progressive muscle weakness and atrophy, muscle fasciculations, spasticity, hyperreflexia, dysphagia, aspiration, dysarthria [4]. Due to severe symptoms and loss of mobility, MND patients require extensive accommodations in surgery. Anesthesia management in these patients is a challenging task because MND patients under anesthesia are at higher risk of respiratory distress, aspiration, and respiratory failure. Thus, anesthetic choices are case-by-case and general guidelines for anesthesia should be adjusted for MND clinical practices.

There are no disease-modifying drugs for ALS. ALS is a rapidly developing disease with an average of few years from diagnosis to death. However, a palliative treatment, Riluzole, can delay ALS progression. Riluzole in combination with stem cell-based therapy may further slow ALS progression [5]. Gene therapy that corrects the *Smn1* gene mutation and thus extends the surviving years for SMA patients was approved by the FDA for children in 2019 [6]. Anesthetic drugs and analgesics could potentially worsen the injury or damage of MND-diseased motor neurons and thus accelerate the disease progression in these patients. Therefore, there are paramount challenges for anesthesiologist to optimize the anesthesia management, post-surgical recoveries and avoid to further damage the motor neurons in MND patients.

2. ALS overview

The underlying etiology of ALS is still unknown but likely multifactorial with the combination of genetic and environmental factors. Approximately 10% of ALS cases exhibit dominant or recessive autosomal transmission of a mutation in the superoxide dismutase gene (SOD-1) [7]. Recent studies reveal that mutations in more than ten genes are possibly involved in the pathogenesis of familial ALS [8].

The initial symptoms of ALS include muscle twitching and weakness in extremities, with difficulty moving, speaking, and swallowing. ALS progresses rapidly, with about 70% of patients dying within 3 years of symptom onset [9]. At the advanced stage of ALS, ALS patients experience respiratory distress and complete paralysis, and requiring ventilatory support and gastrostomy.

In a case report on an ALS patient undergoing open gastrostomy, the choice of epidural anesthesia over general anesthesia was made to avoid possible respiratory complications [10]. The patient, a 56 year-old female with tetraparesis, also had difficulty speaking, and lung opacities possibly due to microaspiration [10]. The patient was determined to suitable for surgery [10]. For the procedure, epidural anesthesia at the T8-9 epidural space with 0.5% levobupivacaine 40 mg and fentanyl 100 μg was followed by sedation with 1% propofol [10]. The operation and post-operative recovery were uneventful [10]. Although neuroaxial anesthesia may incur further damage on motor neurons, it is ideal compared to general anesthesia for prevention of airway manipulation and respiratory complications. Epidural anesthesia allows the titration of local anesthetic and avoids direct contact between the anesthetic and the heightened susceptible spinal cord. The choice of levobupivacaine in this reported case is due to its lessened motor blockade, as well as low neurotoxicity and cardiotoxicity [10]. Thus, the depth of anesthesia should be closely monitored during the entire surgical procedure.

3. Risks of anesthesia in ALS patients

ALS patients are at a high risk of developing hyperkalemia. Succinylcholine administration to ALS patients induces hyperkalemia, resulting in cardiac dysrhythmias and arrest [11]. In another instance, the depolarizing neuromuscular blocking agent suxamethonium chloride triggered catastrophic hyperkalemia in a patient with undiagnosed ALS [12]. Upper and lower motor neuron injuries or denervation in ALS patients lead to the upregulation of nicotinic α7 acetylcholine receptors, the presence of which enables a larger potassium efflux to the bloodstream [13].

Depolarizing neuromuscular blocker can also cause rhabdomyolysis in ALS patients, a serious medical condition that can results in death or permanent disability. Rhabdomyolysis occurs when damaged sarcomeres release a large amount of dysfunctional proteins and electrolytes into circulation. These harmful substances can cause severe injuries to the heart and kidneys [14]. Due to life-threatening hyperkalemia and potential induction of rhabdomyolysis, depolarizing neuromuscular blocks including succinylcholine, an acetylcholine agonist, and suxamethonium chloride should be contraindicated in ALS patients. In the case of non-depolarizing neuromuscular blocking drugs, short-acting drugs should be chosen to avoid adverse effects and should be used in combination with reversal agents to ensure quick recovery from muscle blocking in ALS patients [15]. Carefully controlling the dose of non-depolarizing neuromuscular blocking drugs is needed to avoid prolonged effects and permanent motor neuron damage.

For ALS patients undergoing surgery, careful consideration of the preoperative, intraoperative, and postoperative phases is essential to achieve successful anesthesia without adverse events. Preoperative respiratory function tests such as spirometry [16] and non-invasive ultrasound assessments [17] can be used to predict respiratory distress perioperatively. In spirometry, if the FEV1 (forced expiratory volume in one second)/FVC (forced vital capacity) ratio, also called as the percentage of the FVC expired in one second [18], is lower than 40%, it indicates a high probability of preoperative ventilatory impairment and that general anesthesia is contraindicated. If possible, a complete neurological examination to determine the presence of impaired bulbar functions such as dysphagia and/or dysarthria is critical [19]. ALS patients with bulbar dysfunction should not be premedicated [10].

Preoperative assessment should include patient history, confirmation of ALS diagnosis, chest radiography, arterial blood gas analysis, liver function test, diaphragmatic function test and videofluoroscopy—an x-ray examination of swallowing. After the preoperative assessment on patients' general, bulbar, and respiratory function, the next step is to carefully design preoperative management including premedication and monitoring setup. For premeditation, it is best to avoid opioids. Alternatively, small doses of benzodiazepines. Large doses of benzodiazepines also carry risk of dependence like opioids but to a lesser extent. Prophylaxis against pulmonary aspiration in ALS patients such as a peroral 400 mg dose of cimetidine, an H2-receptor antagonists, should be considered at the preoperative stage.

The next step is to induce and maintain anesthesia in ALS patients and this step depends on the types of chosen anesthesia. For the induction of epidural anesthesia, propofol is used for sedation [10]. In a case of a 63 year-old female ALS patient undergoing open reduction and internal fixation of the right tibia, intravenous administrations of propofol and remifentanil without any muscle relaxants were chosen for the anesthesia method [20]. This anesthetic method effectively avoided the occurrence of ALS exacerbation and ventilatory depression induced by abnormal responses to muscle relaxants [20]. After standard and neuromuscular monitoring devices were placed on the patient without any pre-anesthetic medications, anesthesia was induced by infusing 3 ng/ml remifentanil and 3.0 μg/ml propofol [20]. The maintenance of anesthesia in this patient was achieved by propofol and remifentanil with 100% oxygen [20]. The intubation was successful and the patient was discharged postoperative day 3 [20]. In a 48-year-old male with a 5 year history of ALS, general anesthesia was selected for his laparotomy because of dysphagia and dysarthria [15]. This patient was induced by 80 μg fentanyl and 2 mg/kg of propofol, and 10 mg of rocuronium was administered before endotracheal intubation [15]. Continuous infusion of propofol at 0.05–0.1 mg/kg/min was used for anesthesia maintenance [15]. No additional muscle relaxant was administered to the patient and surgery was successfully completed without any significant sequelae [15]. In the above case, the endotracheal tube was placed prior to anesthesia induction, and extubation was performed with the patient fully awake [15]. For ALS patients, while regional anesthesia is generally a less risky choice than general anesthesia, general anesthesia can be done safely in advanced-stage ALS patients.

4. Propofol and remifentanil in induction and maintenance of anesthesia in ALS patients

For the induction and maintenance of anesthesia in ALS patients, combined propofol and remifentanil are frequently used. Propofol is the most popular intravenous sedation drug. Early pharmacological studies have shown quick whole body distribution and relatively fast clearance [21]. Compared to traditional anesthetics such as barbiturates, thiopental and methohexital, patients under propofol show rapid recovery from anesthesia and significantly lower incidence of postoperative side effects including nausea, vomiting, and cognitive impairment, collectively termed "hang-over effects". Furthermore, patients under propofol exhibit relatively quick recovery in cognitive and psychomotor function [22]. The benefits of propofol also include earlier discharges from the post-anesthesia care unit and higher patient satisfaction for their anesthetic experience [23]. Because of these features, propofol has become the primary choice for an induction agent via intravenous bolus administration and a volatile anesthetic for anesthesia maintenance. With improved drug delivery systems and monitoring, the use of propofol can further benefit high-risk patients such as ALS patients undergoing complex procedures [24].

Remifentanil is a synthetic and short-acting mu-opioid receptor agonist. Other opioids including morphine, fentanyl, alfentanil and sufentanil are also used for pain relief and the use of these opioids is associated with a range of adverse effects. The adverse effects of morphine manifest with histamine release, pruritus, constipation, and the accumulation of metabolite morphine-6-glucuronide in patients with renal impairment [25]. Drug accumulation is a serious concern when opioids are used in surgical procedures. Remifentanil has an ultrashort clearance profile because it can be rapidly metabolized by unspecific blood and tissue esterases [25]. In contrast, fentanyl, alfentanil and sufentanil are all metabolized in the liver. Continuous infusions of these opioids result in drug accumulation and prolonged offset effects. The accumulation of these opioids can cause respiratory depression/failure alongside significantly delayed and unpredictable recovery in ALS patients. The simultaneous use of remifentanil and propofol has unique beneficial effects. Studies comparing the sedative effect of these two drugs in regional anesthesia have demonstrated that remifentanil is more effective than propofol in decreasing pain but has a higher incidence of nausea and respiratory depression [26, 27]. A study on combining propofol or midazolam with either sufentanil or remifentanil reveals that either <3 mg/kg/h propofol, 0.5–3 mg/h midazolam with 5–10 μg/h sufentanil, or 0.05 μg/kg/min remifentanil can achieve successful sedation in regional blocks with a low incidence of adverse events [28]. Further studies in using different administration methods identify that a bolus administration for induction along with continuous infusion of propofol for maintenance is ideal for successful sedation and quick recovery [29]. It has been shown that remifentanil is associated with development of hyperalgesia in patients [30]. However, propofol infusion decreases the incidence of remifentanil-induced hyperalgesia [31]. Therefore, the combination of remifentanil and propofol can overcome the adverse effects of remifentanil including respiratory depression and nausea while keeping the advantage of remifentanil in effectively blocking pain during surgeries. This method should be recommended for ALS patients undergoing either regional or general anesthesia.

5. Intraoperative nondepolarizing neuromuscular blockers in ALS patients

While depolarizing neuromuscular blockers are contraindicated, nondepolarizing neuromuscular blockers such as rocuronium has been successfully used along with propofol and remifentanil. In a case of a 47 year-old ALS patient with a humerus fracture, general anesthesia was induced by propofol, rocuronium and remifentanil [32]. At the end of an uneventful operation, TOF (train-of-four) was great than 0.90 but muscle strengthen and tidal volume were not sufficient [32]. Rocuronium and other nondepolarizing neuromuscular blockers are competitive antagonists of the post-synaptic acetylcholine receptor, leading to prolonged weakness or flaccid paralysis. In the above case, 2 mg/kg sugammadex was given intravenously to quench the residual remifentanil in the patient [32]. Suggammadex rapidly forms a complex with free rocuronium, which is quickly filtered by the kidney. Thus, the duo of rocuronium and sugammadex has been frequently and safely used in general anesthesia of ALS patients.

6. Postoperative care for ALS patients

Tracheal extubation should be done after the patient is fully awake. This will maximize the laryngeal reflex function. Regardless, the respiratory status of the patient needs be closely monitored. In some cases, postoperative ventilation is needed, and weaning ventilation should be prolonged. Patients who had noninvasive positive-pressure ventilation (NPPV) preoperatively require NPPV being placed once again postoperatively [33]. There is a need for effective pain relief but the use of agents that depress respiration should be avoided. It is recommended to use peripheral nerve blockers and local or regional approaches to manage postoperative pain. Postoperative oxygen use is not recommended due to the instability of respiratory control in ALS patients. When opioids are used, the dosages should be tightly controlled in conjunction with monitoring methods such as pulse oximetry to reduce morbidity and mortality.

In case of an ALS patient with rectal cancer, laparoscopic low anterior resection with diverting loop ileostomy and total abdominal hysterectomy were performed under general anesthesia using the combination of propofol and rocuronium for induction and the regime of sevoflurane and remifentanil for maintenance [34]. After the surgery, glycopyrrolate and pyridostigmine bromide were used to reverse the muscle relaxant effects of rocuronium [34]. Postoperative use of fentanyl controlling analgesia in the patient consisted of intermittent low doses within 48 hours, and the patient recovered uneventfully [34]. The use of fentanyl should be cautioned against as it causes respiratory muscle rigidity and subsequent respiratory dysfunction in ALS patients. Postoperative pain should be carefully managed based on the unique circumstances of ALS patients.

7. Anesthesia during labor and delivery in ALS patients

Because ALS onset is usually late in life, there are few cases associated with labor and delivery in ALS patients. How pregnancy affects the progression of ALS is still unclear. It has been reported that ALS patients have successfully carried pregnancies to term [35]. The timing and the methods of delivery are chosen based on the disease stage. The perineum and the uterine musculature are not affected by ALS, and thus vaginal delivery is a preferred method for labor. Progressive shortness of breath or respiratory distress during pregnancy are indicators for emergency Caesarean section [35]. ALS patients are often unable to increase respiration to match oxygen need in labor. As respiratory burden worsens at the end of pregnancy, anesthetic management during Caesarean section becomes increasingly challenging.

There is no formal recommendation for anesthesia management of Caesarean section in women with ALS. It has been reported that epidural anesthesia has been used successfully with no evidence of anesthesia complications in ALS patients. In a case of 38-week pregnant woman with 10-year history of ALS, sequential combined spinal-epidural anesthesia was successful for Caesarean section [36]. Before delivery, neurological assessment on the patient showed progressive muscle weakness, severe dysarthria and dysphagia. The patient presented with quadriparesis, hypotonia, and hyperreflexia, and severe restriction on spirometry with a high risk of respiratory failure. Prior to anesthesia, doses of ranitidine, metoclopramide and dexamethasone are given. Hyperbaric bupivacaine 6 mg plus fentanyl 10 μg were given through the spinal needle and 5 minute later with 0.25% isobaric bupivacaine in 10 ml through the epidural catheter to block T5. The surgical procedure was uneventful. Thus, while vaginal delivery is ideal, delicate regional anesthesia can achieve good outcomes for Caesarean section.

8. SMA overview

SMA is a spectrum of MNDs occurring predominantly in infants and children. The primary causal factors for this inherited disease are deletions or mutations of the *Smn1* gene. Generally, *Smn1* gene deficiency causes the degeneration and eventual death of spinal anterior horn neurons with decreased brainstem nuclei. SMA type I (Werdnig-Hoffmann) shows symptoms before 6 months of age and progresses rapidly in the first year of life. SMA types II and III (Kugelberg-Welander) manifest at 6–18 months of age and later in childhood, respectively. SMA type 0, the most severe and earliest onset form, is fatal without respiratory support. The symptoms of SMA type IV first appear in adulthood, presenting with minimal disability.

Infants and children with SMA often need anesthesia because of diagnostic procedures and surgical treatments. Common procedures associated with SMA type I patients are gastrostomy, fundoplication, tracheotomy, and muscle biopsy. Common procedures for SMA type II and III patients include correction of scoliosis and club foot, joint contracture release, and muscle biopsy. SMA type III patients can reach reproductive age and thus cesarean sections may be performed on these patients.

9. Anesthetic management of SMA patients

SMA patients have prominent spinal and other bone deformities that require surgical correction to improve patients' quality of life and extend their survival time. In a case of a 14-year-old SMA type II male patient with a previous operation for scoliosis, the patient was scheduled for an implant removal because of infection [37]. General anesthesia was used and 2 mg dormicum, 20 mg lidocaine, 80 mg propofol, 25 μg fentanyl were used for the induction of anesthesia [37]. No neuromuscular blockers were used [37]. The patient was intubated with a spiral cuffed number 5 tube with direct laryngoscopy when his Bispectral Index Score, which monitors consciousness, was 46 [37]. Foe anesthesia maintenance, one percent sevoflurane and remifentanyl infusion of 0.1–0.2 mg/kg/min were used [37]. The surgery was uneventful and an intravenous administration of 25 mg dexketoprofen was given for postoperative analgesia [37]. The patient was successfully extubated and followed up in intensive care for one day postoperatively [37]. As in this case study, general anesthesia for major surgery in SMA patients should be performed using minimal opioids, whereas muscle blockers are to be used judiciously. Combining sevoflurane with remifentanil, which quickly reverses the muscle relaxant effect of sevoflurane, can achieve optimal anesthesia management and postoperative recovery.

Likewise, there are two cases of general anesthesia for surgical correction of heart defects in SMA type II patients [38]. A 23-day-old SMA type 2 patient successfully underwent pulmonary banding and patent ductus arteriosus ligation with 4 mg thiopental, 4 mg fentanyl, and 1.5 mg rocuronium being used for anesthesia induction and maintenance [38]. Atrial and ventricular septal defect closure and pulmonary artery reconstruction were performed on a 17-month-old patient using rocuronium, pentothal, dormicum, and fentanyl, with maintenance via 0.1 mg/kg/h precedex and 0.6–0.7 minimum alveolar concentration (MAC) of sevoflurane [38]. Both patients were extubated and recovered uneventfully [38].

In a case of an 8 year-old SMA type II patient, a dislocated hip was corrected with a combination general and local anesthesia regimen [39]. Similar to the aforementioned cases, the patient was induced by sevoflurane followed by intravenous administration of fentanyl and propofol [39]. Spinal anesthesia was achieved with 2 ml 0.5% hyperbaric bupivacaine with an epidural catheter in the L3–L4 space [39]. The patient successfully recovered.

Graham *et al*. summarizes anesthesia induction and management for 56 cases of SMA types I, II and III [40]. Midazolam via both enteral and intravenous routes or a combination of ketamine and midazolam were used for premedication [40]. The most common method for airway support is standard endotracheal intubation. Propofol-based intravenous anesthesia is the most common approach during the procedure. Cisatracurium is the first line neuromuscular blocker, while fentanyl and remifentanil are the two most commonly used intraoperative opioids.

10. SMA patient perioperative care essentials

In a retrospective chart study, thoracolumbar spinal deformity corrections were performed in 34 SMA type I and II patients in a single medical center from 1990 to 2015 [41]. The study reported that in the 34 patients, there were two occurrences of pneumonia (6%), no postoperative re-intubation or unplanned tracheostomies, and no deaths [41]. Because SMA is associated with impaired gastrointestinal function and malnutrition, most SMA patients need perioperative total parenteral nutrition (TPN), whichbypasses the gastrointestinal tract and delivers nutrients to the venous system. Additionally, these patients must be on continuous NPPV for adequate respiratory support.

Pulmonary disease and bulbar dysfunction are strongly associated with SMA and pose anesthetic risks. Preoperatively, pulmonary consultation should be done in all SMA patients. Pulmonary function tests should be conducted. Most SMA patients have difficulties with intubation and thorough evaluations on indicators for intubation should be considered. Preoperative training on NIPPV should be conducted if the patient currently does not have respiratory support. Preoperative airway evaluation is mandatory and establishes a plan for intubation difficulties due to. SMA patients are susceptible for to hypo- and hyperglycemia. Thus, blood glucose levels should be closely monitored. Cardiac function needs to be evaluated preoperatively because SMA is often associated with cardiac malformations. SMA type I and II patients often have gastroesophageal reflux and should be evaluated accordingly.

Intraoperatively, endotracheal intubation with positive pressure ventilation should be applied as respiratory support. Depolarizing muscle relaxants such as succinylcholine should be constrained and the dose of nondepolarizing muscle relaxants should be tightly controlled. If nondepolarizing muscle relaxants are used, neuromuscular function should be monitored. Inhaled anesthetics should be avoided in favor of the intravenous route. Short acting opioids are used intra-operatively when opioids are needed. TPN infusion should be maintained to avoid hypoglycemia. SMA patients typically have 2 more hours of anesthetic time than healthy patients.

Postoperatively, SMA patients should be monitored in the intensive care unit. Generally, these patients require 5–7 days of intensive care even with minor procedures. Most SMA type I patients need postoperative ventilatory support. Postoperative oxygen supplementation is needed for the first 24 hours. Opioids, acetaminophen, and NSAIDs, or all three in combination should be used as postoperative pain management. Opioids may induce respiratory distress in SMA patients. Benzodiazepines are used to manage muscle spasms and discomfort. However, postoperative pain management can largely be tailored to the individual.

11. Kennedy's disease overview and anesthetic management

Kennedy's disease (KD), also known as spinal and bulbar muscular atrophy, is a rare adulthood-onset X-linked disease that results in the degeneration and eventual death of lower motor neurons. The major symptoms of KD are tongue atrophy, dysarthria, dysphonia and dysphagia, along with limb and bulbar muscle atrophy, weakness and fasciculations [42]. KD is a CAG trinucleotide expansion repeat disorder in the androgen receptor gene. Anesthetic management can be challenging. Laryngospasm and pulmonary aspiration have been reported as primary anesthetic risks in KD patients. Both nondepolarizing and depolarizing neuromuscular blockers induce hyperkalemia in KD patients [42]. In a 71-year old KD male patient who underwent a tracheotomy, the surgical procedure was performed under local anesthesia by ultrasound-guided superior laryngeal nerve block and superficial cervical plexus block via 2% lidocaine [42]. The procedure was uneventful and the patient reported no discomfort [42]. In a 61-year-old male KD patient who underwent a left thigh sarcoma excision, general anesthesia with endotracheal intubation was induced by 150 mg propofol and 100 μg fentanyl, and maintained with inhalational anesthesia [43]. The patient recovered without any postoperative complications.

12. Isaacs' syndrome overview and anesthetic management

Isaacs' syndrome, a peripheral MND, manifests with peripheral nerve hyperexcitability. Symptoms include cramps, muscle stiffness, muscle twitching, and pseudomyotonia. The major cause of Isaacs' syndrome is antibodies against the voltage-gated potassium channel complex in the peripheral nerves. Anticonvulsive medications and immunomodulation therapy are used to control the progression of this disease. The onset of Isaacs' syndrome is mainly in early adulthood or onwards.

In a 74-year-old female Isaacs' syndrome patient who underwent a surgery for open rotator cuff repair, total intravenous anesthesia with propofol, remifentanil, and atracurium was used under continuous neuromuscular monitoring [44]. The surgical procedure and postoperative recovery were smooth without any anesthetic complications. Because Isaacs' syndrome is a rare disorder, anesthetic management and outcomes have not been extensively explored in literature.

Conflict of interest statement

The authors have declared that no conflict of interest exists

Declaration of interests

The author declares no competing interests.

Author details

Wendy Wenqiao Yang
Morsani College of Medicine, University of South Florida, Tampa, FL, USA

*Address all correspondence to: wendyyang@usf.edu

References

[1] Kiernan MC et al. Amyotrophic lateral sclerosis. Lancet. 2011;**377**:942-955

[2] Shababi M, Lorson CL, Rudnik-Schoneborn SS. Spinal muscular atrophy: A motor neuron disorder or a multi-organ disease? Journal of Anatomy. 2014;**224**:15-28

[3] Park J, Kim JE, Song TJ. The global burden of motor neuron disease: An analysis of the 2019 global burden of disease study. Frontiers in Neurology. 2022;**13**:864339

[4] Mei XW et al. Identifying key signs of motor neurone disease in primary care: A nested case-control study using the QResearch database. BMJ Open. 2022;**12**:e058383

[5] Abdul Wahid SF, Law ZK, Ismail NA, Lai NM. Cell-based therapies for amyotrophic lateral sclerosis/motor neuron disease. Cochrane Database of Systematic Reviews. 2019;**12**:CD011742

[6] Ali HG et al. Gene therapy for spinal muscular atrophy: The Qatari experience. Gene Therapy. 2021;**28**:676-680

[7] Battistini S et al. SOD1 mutations in amyotrophic lateral sclerosis. Results from a multicenter Italian study. Journal of Neurology. 2005;**252**:782-788

[8] Siddique T, Ajroud-Driss S. Familial amyotrophic lateral sclerosis, a historical perspective. Acta Myologica. 2011;**30**:117-120

[9] Walling AD. Amyotrophic lateral sclerosis: Lou Gehrig's disease. American Family Physician. 1999;**59**:1489-1496

[10] Ruiz-Chirosa MDC et al. Epidural anesthesia for open gastrostomy in a patient with amyotrophic lateral sclerosis. Colombian Journal of Anesthesiology. 2018;**46**:246-249

[11] Giaovanni JA. Anesthesia complications in the dental office. In: Bosack RC, Lieblich S, editors. Anesthetic Considertion for Patients with Neurologic Disease. 1st ed. John Wiley & Sons, Inc.; 2015. pp. 79-84

[12] Turner MR, Lawrence H, Arnold I, Ansorge O, Talbot K. Catastrophic hyperkalaemia following administration of suxamethonium chloride to a patient with undiagnosed amyotrophic lateral sclerosis. Clinical Medicine (London, England). 2011;**11**:292-293

[13] Hovgaard HL, Juhl-Olsen P. Suxamethonium-induced hyperkalemia: A short review of causes and recommendations for clinical applications. Critical Care Research and Practice. 2021;**2021**:6613118

[14] Torres PA, Helmstetter JA, Kaye AM, Kaye AD. Rhabdomyolysis: Pathogenesis, diagnosis, and treatment. The Ochsner Journal. 2015;**15**:58-69

[15] Sarna R, Gupta A, Arora G. Amyotrophic lateral sclerosis and anaesthetic challenges: Perioperative lignocaine infusion-an aid. Indian Journal of Anaesthesia. 2020;**64**:448-449

[16] Fallat RJ, Jewitt B, Bass M, Kamm B, Norris FH Jr. Spirometry in amyotrophic lateral sclerosis. Archives of Neurology. 1979;**36**:74-80

[17] Fantini R et al. Serial ultrasound assessment of diaphragmatic function and clinical outcome in patients with

amyotrophic lateral sclerosis. BMC Pulmonary Medicine. 2019;**19**:160

[18] Barreiro TJ, Perillo I. An approach to interpreting spirometry. American Family Physician. 2004;**69**:1107-1114

[19] Prabhakar A, Owen CP, Kaye AD. Anesthetic management of the patient with amyotrophic lateral sclerosis. Journal of Anesthesia. 2013;**27**:909-918

[20] Lee D, Lee KC, Kim JY, Park YS, Chang YJ. Total intravenous anesthesia without muscle relaxant in a patient with amyotrophic lateral sclerosis. Journal of Anesthesia. 2008;**22**:443-445

[21] Shafer A, Doze VA, Shafer SL, White PF. Pharmacokinetics and pharmacodynamics of propofol infusions during general anesthesia. Anesthesiology. 1988;**69**:348-356

[22] Doze VA, Westphal LM, White PF. Comparison of propofol with methohexital for outpatient anesthesia. Anesthesia and Analgesia. 1986;**65**:1189-1195

[23] Tang J et al. Recovery profile, costs, and patient satisfaction with propofol and sevoflurane for fast-track office-based anesthesia. Anesthesiology. 1999;**91**:253-261

[24] White PF. Propofol: Its role in changing the practice of anesthesia. Anesthesiology. 2008;**109**:1132-1136

[25] Wilhelm W, Kreuer S. The place for short-acting opioids: Special emphasis on remifentanil. Critical Care. 2008;**12**(Suppl 3):S5

[26] Mingus ML, Monk TG, Gold MI, Jenkins W, Roland C. Remifentanil versus propofol as adjuncts to regional anesthesia. Remifentanil 3010 Study Group. Journal of Clinical Anesthesia. 1998;**10**:46-53

[27] Servin FS et al. Remifentanil sedation compared with propofol during regional anaesthesia. Acta Anaesthesiologica Scandinavica. 2002;**46**:309-315

[28] Savoia G et al. Monitored anesthesia care and loco-regional anesthesia. Vascular surgery use. Minerva Anestesiol. 2005;**71**:539-542

[29] Hohener D, Blumenthal S, Borgeat A. Sedation and regional anaesthesia in the adult patient. British Journal of Anaesthesia. 2008;**100**:8-16

[30] Schmidt S, Bethge C, Forster MH, Schafer M. Enhanced postoperative sensitivity to painful pressure stimulation after intraoperative high dose remifentanil in patients without significant surgical site pain. The Clinical Journal of Pain. 2007;**23**:605-611

[31] Singler B, Troster A, Manering N, Schuttler J, Koppert W. Modulation of remifentanil-induced postinfusion hyperalgesia by propofol. Anesthesia and Analgesia. 2007;**104**:1397-1403, table of contents

[32] Kelsaka E, Karakaya D, Zengin EC. Use of sugammadex in a patient with amyotrophic lateral sclerosis. Medical Principles and Practice. 2013;**22**:304-306

[33] Onders RP et al. Amyotrophic lateral sclerosis: The Midwestern surgical experience with the diaphragm pacing stimulation system shows that general anesthesia can be safely performed. American Journal of Surgery. 2009;**197**:386-390

[34] Kim B-R, Lee Y-B, Kim S-J, Kim Y-W. Anesthetic considerations for laparoscopy for rectal cancer in patient with amyotrophic lateral sclerosis: A case report. Egyptian Journal of Anaesthesia. 2018;**34**:175-176

[35] Pathiraja PDM, Ranaraja SK. A successful pregnancy with amyotrophic lateral sclerosis. Case Reports in Obstetrics and Gynecology. 2020;**2020**:1247178

[36] Moreno-Gonzales R, Vásquez-Rojas G, Rojas Fun M. Anaesthetic management of a patient diagnosed with amyotrophic lateral sclerosis taken to caesarean section: Case report. Colombian Journal of Anesthesiology. 2017;**45**:86-89

[37] Akcaalan Y, Erkilic E, Akin M. Anesthesia management in patient with spinal muscular atrophy (SMA) type 2. American Journal of Surgery and Clinical Case Reports. 2022;**4**:1-3

[38] Bicer M, Kozan S, Ozturk F, Akcay AA. Surgical correction of a ventricular septal defect in a child with spinal muscular atrophy type 2 treated with nusinersen sodium: A case report. Journal of Cardiothoracic Surgery. 2023;**18**:68

[39] Panda S, Baby SKR, Singh G. Spinal muscular atrophy type II: Anesthetic challenges and perioperative management. Journal of Cardiac Critical Care TSS. 2021;**05**:249-251

[40] Graham RJ, Athiraman U, Laubach AE, Sethna NF. Anesthesia and perioperative medical management of children with spinal muscular atrophy. Paediatric Anaesthesia. 2009;**19**:1054-1063

[41] Halanski MA et al. Peri-operative management of children with spinal muscular atrophy. Indian Journal of Anaesthesia. 2020;**64**:931-936

[42] Colizza A et al. Anesthetic and surgical management of tracheotomy in a patient with Kennedy's disease. La Clinica Terapeutica. 2022;**173**:503-506

[43] Evans R, Escher AR Jr, Nahrwold DA, Hoffman JP. General anesthesia with successful immediate post-operative extubation for sarcoma excision in a 61-year-old male with Kennedy's disease. Cureus. 2022;**14**:e21956

[44] Kim YM et al. Anesthetic experience using total intravenous anesthesia in a patient with Isaacs' syndrome - A case report. Korean Journal of Anesthesiology. 2013;**64**:164-167

Chapter 6

Acupuncture Treatment for Dystonia

Makiko Tani and Toshiaki Suzuki

Abstract

This article introduces acupuncture for dystonia, especially cervical dystonia and upper limb dystonia. In our acupuncture treatment, the meridians corresponding to the affected muscles are identified, and stimulation of the acupuncture points located on the meridians away from the affected muscles is used. Affected muscles may have problems of hypotonia as well as hypertonia. We will introduce a method of suppressing muscle tone using acupuncture points and a method of promoting muscle tone. Furthermore, since shortening of muscles and skin may affect posture abnormalities and movement abnormalities, we will also introduce the treatment. This article presents a case for our therapeutic effect.

Keywords: cervical dystonia, upper extremity dystonia, acupuncture treatment, acupuncture points, electromyography

1. Introduction

Dystonia is defined as "a syndrome of sustained muscle contractions, frequently causing twisting and repetitive movements, or abnormal postures" and is considered a syndrome of dyskinesia rather than a disease. It can be classified as generalized, segmental, or focal, depending on the affected region. Cervical dystonia and upper extremity dystonia, which are discussed in this paper, are localized dystonia. Focal dystonia is reported to occur in 3 to 38 per 100,000 population [1]. The cause is often unknown, but hereditary dystonia involving genetic abnormalities has been identified. It has been hypothesized that focal dystonia may be triggered by frequent use of the neck or upper extremities, but it is not known if such activity is an obvious cause.

The current first choice for medical treatment is botulinum therapy. Other non-surgical treatments include transcranial magnetic stimulation, biofeedback, and psychotherapy. In addition, oral medications such as anticholinergics are used as adjuncts. When these non-surgical treatments are not effective, surgery may be performed. Surgical procedures include deep brain stimulation (DBS), selective thalamotomy, and parasympathetic decompression surgery.

Acupuncture may be useful as a non-surgical treatment for dystonia, but there have been only a few scattered reports of acupuncture for dystonia.

The authors have been treating dystonia with acupuncture since 1995. Currently, botulinum therapy is considered the first-line treatment for dystonia. Other standard treatments include DBS, stereotactic brain surgery, and oral medication. Acupuncture, on the other hand, is not often considered an option. We have used acupuncture to treat patients whose symptoms have not improved after botulinum toxin therapy and oral medications. In this paper, we introduce the method of acupuncture treatment and our thoughts on the treatment [2–4].

2. Introduction to acupuncture treatment

For the benefit of our readers, we feel it necessary to first introduce acupuncture. The acupuncture treatment that the authors are using is Japanese-style acupuncture needles. The needles are made of stainless steel and are disposable. The needles we use are 0.2 mm in diameter, which are much thinner than injection needles. Regarding the area to be treated, botulinum treatment or alcohol blockade would involve injecting a chemical solution into the affected muscle that is hypertonic. In our acupuncture treatment, we use acupuncture points as the target of treatment. The acupuncture points have an important meaning in acupuncture treatment. However, their actual status has not been confirmed anatomically. In this regard, it is not surprising that a non-acupuncturist would question the significance of acupuncture in medicine. However, in the 1990s and 2000s, there was a growing awareness of Oriental medicine in terms of complementary and alternative medicine (CAM) and integrative medicine. In 2003, the WHO began to consider international acupuncture point location standardization as part of its work to standardize acupuncture terminology, and in 2008, the WHO/WPRO: WHO Western Pacific Region Office published the "WHO Standard Acupuncture Point Locations in the Western Pacific Region" [5]. In this text, 14 meridians and 361 acupuncture points are summarized. We use this concept of meridians and acupuncture points in acupuncture treatment for dystonia to regulate muscle tone in the affected muscles.

3. Acupuncture treatment for cervical dystonia

In cervical dystonia, the sternocleidomastoid, splenius, and trapezius (upper fibers) muscles are considered typical affected muscles. When improving the muscle tone of each affected muscle with acupuncture, there are some points to keep in mind. One of the hypothesized mechanisms of dystonia is to normalize the "abnormality in the motor subroutine formed by sensory input and motor output" [6]. Therefore, the acupuncture needle insertion depth is made shallow, 0.5 mm or less, to make the stimulation milder and to normalize sensory input through stimulation of the cutaneous nerves.

3.1 Evaluation of changes in cervical muscle tone using surface electromyography

We present the effects of acupuncture treatment on a case of cervical dystonia with left lateral flexion-right rotation deviation of the neck (Case 1) (**Table 1**). In the prone position, surface electromyography of the bilateral sternocleidomastoid muscles and bilateral upper trapezius muscle fibers was recorded. As a result, a marked increase in muscle activity was observed in the left upper trapezius muscle fibers. Acupuncture was performed using stainless steel disposable needles (0.2 mm in diameter) placed at a depth of 5 mm into the left Bailao (Ex-HN15), an acupuncture point located on the left upper trapezius muscle fiber. After the

	Gender	Age	Medical diagnosis	Interventions	Therapeutic effects
Case 1	male	36	cervical dystonia	acupuncture MAB* medication	effective no effect supplementary effect
Case 2	female	68	cervical dystonia	acupuncture medication	effective supplementary effect
Case 3	female	21	cervical dystonia	acupuncture medication	effective no effect
Case 4	male	44	upper limb dystonia	acupuncture MAB* Medication orthopedic therapy	effective slightly effect supplementary effect no effect

**MAB: muscle afferent block.*

Table 1.
Background of the patients.

acupuncture treatment, muscle activity of the left upper trapezius muscle fibers decreased. Treatment was continued at weekly intervals, and after approximately 5 months, no abnormal activity was observed on the surface electromyogram in the supine position (**Figure 1**). However, in the sitting and standing positions, cervical deviation remained, and re-evaluation of the surface EMG in the sitting position revealed increased muscle activity in both the bilateral sternocleido-mastoid and bilateral upper trapezius fibers (**Figure 2**). The same treatment was continued, and the patient no longer showed abnormalities in the surface EMG waveforms in the sitting position. This confirmed the importance of considering the treatment posture during acupuncture treatment.

3.2 Effects of treatment on remote acupuncture points

As mentioned above, it was confirmed that treatment to acupuncture points located above the affected muscle was effective. Next, we examined the effect of acupuncture treatment on meridians located at sites other than on the affected muscles. In Oriental medicine and acupuncture and moxibustion treatment, the meridians that pass through the site of the patient's symptoms are identified, and the acupuncture points belonging to these meridians are considered to be the treatment sites. The acupuncture point to be treated may be set at a remote location, not at the site of the symptoms. In the acupuncture treatment for cervical dystonia, the meridian running over the affected muscle was identified, and the acupuncture points on that meridian but distant from the affected muscle were used as the treatment site.

In a patient with cervical left lateral flexion-right rotation deviation (Case 2), a surface electromyogram was recorded, confirming increased muscle tone in the left upper trapezius muscle fibers. We then selected the left Waiguan (TE5) from the Triple Energizer meridian, which is a meridian that passes over the upper trapezius muscle fibers, and placed acupuncture needles on the left Waiguan (TE5). As a result, the peak-to-peak amplitude and mean rectified voltage of the surface electromyogram decreased with each passing minute, immediately after the needles were removed (POST 0), 5 minutes later (POST 5), and 10 minutes after (POST 10) the needles were removed, compared to before treatment, and improvement in neck posture was also observed (**Figure 3**). Such a phenomenon of a decrease in muscle tone over time

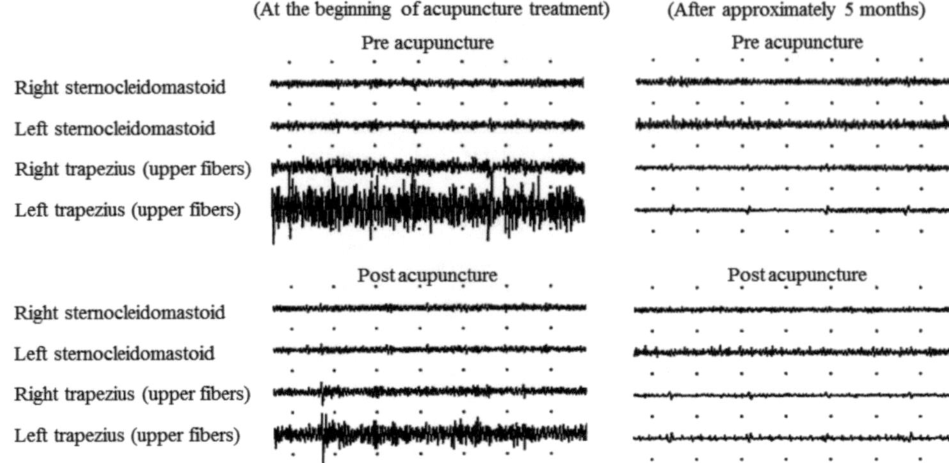

Figure 1.
Long-term acupuncture treatment significantly reduced the abnormal muscle activity seen in each test muscle before acupuncture treatment. The effect of acupuncture treatment was pronounced when abnormal muscle activity was observed before acupuncture treatment. However, when no abnormal muscle activity was observed before acupuncture treatment, almost no change was observed.

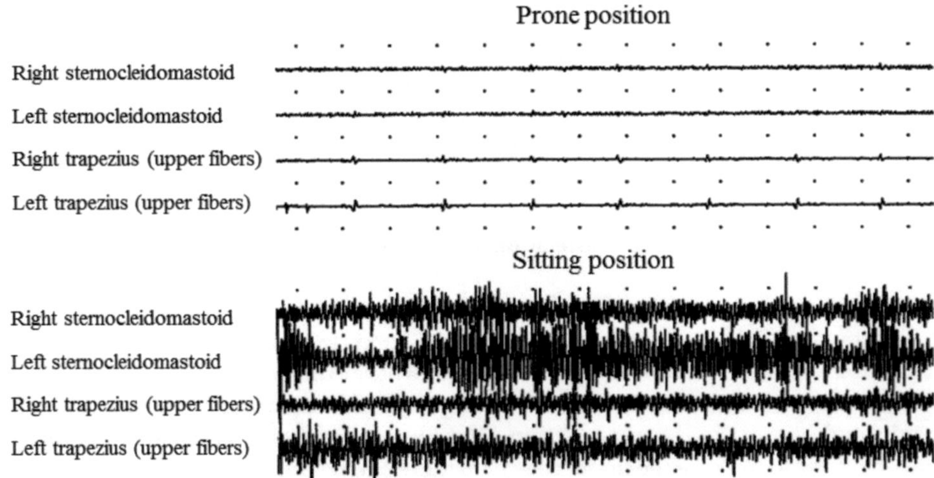

Figure 2.
Surface EMG waveform changes with postural changes on the same examination day are shown. No abnormal EMG activity was observed in each examined muscle in the prone position, but in the sitting position, abnormal EMG activity was prominent.

even after the needles were removed was not observed when the acupuncture points on the affected muscles were used as the treatment sites. These results indicate that acupuncture treatment at acupuncture points belonging to meridians running over the affected muscle and located remotely from the affected muscle is effective.

3.3 Therapeutic acupuncture points for affected muscles of cervical dystonia

After having treated the abnormal muscle tone of the upper trapezius muscle with the Waiguan (TE5) of the Triple Energizer meridian, we set up treatment acupoints

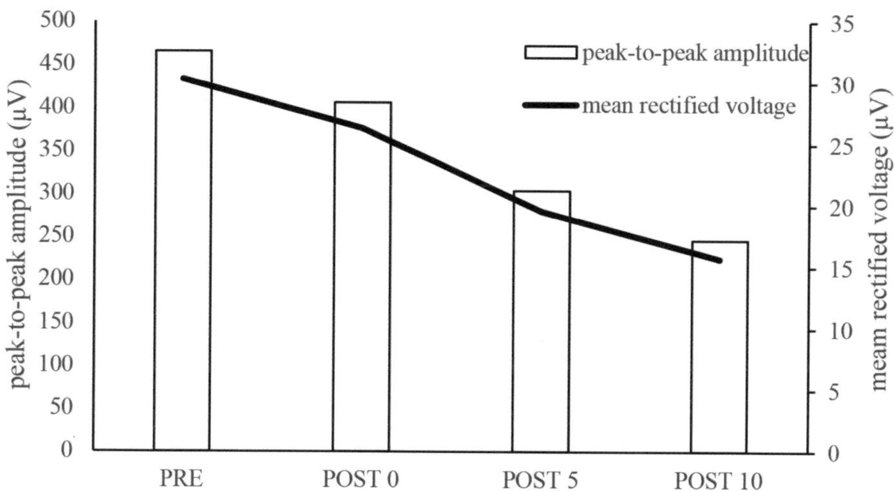

Figure 3.
Left trapezius EMG changes before and after stimulation of the left Waiguan (TE5).

for the other affected muscles. For the sternocleidomastoid muscle, we used Hegu (LI4) of the Large Intestine meridian, and for the splenius muscle, we used Houxi (SI3) of the Small Intestine meridian or the Waiguan (TE5) of the Triple Energizer meridian. In addition, Kunlun (BL60) of the Bladder meridian is used for the levator scapulae muscle, and Chongyang (ST42) of the Stomach meridian is used for the oblique muscles. Furthermore, even in cases of cervical dystonia, the affected muscles that affect cervical bias may not be limited to the cervical muscles. For example, in cases of cervical retroversion, which is often difficult to treat, there may be decreased tone in the abdominal muscles and increased tone in the dorsal muscles in addition to cervical muscle problems. In this case, one can use the Stomach meridian, Chongyang (ST42) for the abdominal muscle group and the Bladder meridian, Kunlun (BL60) for the dorsal muscle group.

3.4 Setting the duration of acupuncture placement in adjusting muscle tone in affected muscles

In general, the problem of dystonia is often thought of as hypertonia of the affected muscles. In fact, the standard treatment with botulinum therapy, alcohol blocks, and oral medications is thought to be aimed at decreasing hypertonia. However, the muscles affected by dystonia may show not only hypertonia but also hypotonia, which is described as "negative dystonia". For example, a surface electromyography study of a patient with left cervical rotation deviation may show no muscle activity in the right sternocleidomastoid muscle at rest. Furthermore, the left sternocleidomastoid muscle may not be fully engaged as the primary active muscle when the patient is asked to perform a right cervical rotation movement. In such cases, suppressing muscle tone in the right sternocleidomastoid muscle as a problem of left cervical rotation deflection does not lead to improvement of cervical posture. Therefore, treatment for decreased muscle tone should be considered.

We experienced an event in which we were able to increase muscle tone during acupuncture treatment of a patient. The patient had a left lateral flexion-right rotation bias of the neck (Case 3). We treated the affected muscle, the left sternocleidomastoid

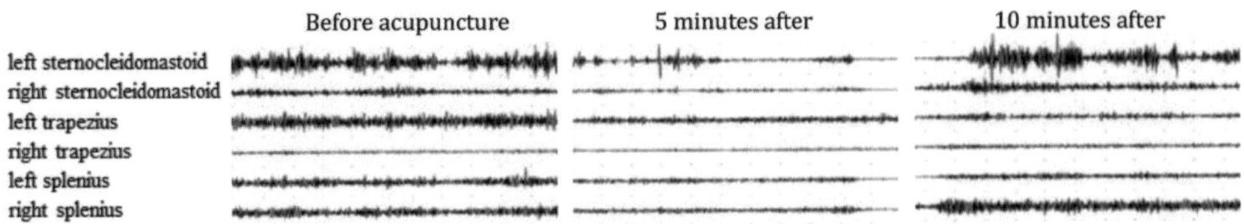

Figure 4.
The electromyographic waveform of the left sternocleidomastoid muscle was inhibited at 5 minutes after acupuncture stimulation and facilitated at 10 minutes after stimulation to left Hegu (LI4).

by left Hegu (LI4), and observed changes in muscle activity using surface electromyography. Five minutes after the start of acupuncture stimulation, the muscle tone of the left sternocleidomastoid muscle was suppressed, but after following the time course, muscle activity of the left sternocleidomastoid muscle was observed again 10 minutes after the start of acupuncture stimulation (**Figure 4**). From this result, we considered that prolonging the duration of acupuncture stimulation could increase muscle tone. Thereafter, the stimulation time was shortened for the purpose of suppressing muscle tone and lengthened for the purpose of facilitating muscle tone. The standard duration of stimulation is from 5 minutes until muscle tone inhibition is confirmed and from 10 minutes until muscle tone stimulation is confirmed in the case of muscle tone stimulation. At this point, it is important to determine the exact point at which the effect is obtained since the time of effect differs depending on the affected muscle. In addition, as mentioned above, the same acupuncture points are used to treat one affected muscle for both muscle tone control to inhibit and facilitate. Therefore, it is even more important to confirm the stimulation time.

3.5 Acupuncture treatment for involuntary movements

Cervical dystonia requires treatment of the affected muscles. Along with this, treatment of involuntary movements is often necessary. In such cases, we treat the affected muscles that produce involuntary movements and simultaneously apply acupuncture to the acupuncture point on the head, Baihui (GV20). In Oriental medicine, it is believed that "wind" is responsible for involuntary movements. Baihui (GV20) is considered to be an acupuncture point to treat diseases that bring about "wind," and it is also effective in treating involuntary movements in dystonia. The needles used are 0.2 mm in diameter, and the depth of penetration is 5 mm or less, as with the acupuncture points for the affected muscles. The duration of stimulation should be determined by checking the degree of suppression of involuntary movements.

3.6 Dealing with muscle shortening and skin shortening

The primary disability brought about by dystonia is abnormal muscle tone and involuntary movements. However, if the affected muscles are in a state of persistent contraction, or if some muscles are inactive because of persistence of the same cervical bias, a secondary disorder may result in muscle shortening and skin shortening. In this case, in addition to acupuncture to the acupuncture points, the muscle shortening or skin shortening should be stretched. We use acupuncture needles that can be stimulated from the skin surface or stretched manually on the shortened skin or muscles. The acupuncture needles used to stimulate the skin from the skin surface are called "syu-mou-shin," which are used in Japan to treat children and are used to stimulate the shortened area while stretching it.

4. Acupuncture treatment for upper extremity dystonia

Typical symptoms of upper extremity dystonia include writer's cramp and musician's cramp. Other cases may cause involuntary movements or abnormalities in muscle activity that impair the movements of those who perform the same movements repeatedly in their occupations.

In these cases, as with cervical dystonia, we identify the affected muscles and treat with consideration of the meridians and acupoints. When treating patients with upper limb symptoms, it is important to consider the relationship of the symptoms to the trunk muscles. For example, in a case of writer's cramp, when the patient's hand trembles and writing is difficult, the problem may be limited to the forearm or hand muscles. However, sufficient muscle activity of the serratus anterior and anterior deltoid fibers is necessary to coordinate upper extremity movements. It is also necessary to check for normal activity of the trunk and buttock muscles to maintain a sitting posture.

In the treatment of upper extremity dystonia, there is a distinctive treatment area. This is the "upper-limb area" proposed by Seikichi Wada. It is a 2 cm straight line drawn from the front one-third of the area that divides the temporal hairline into three equal parts toward the top of the head. In the treatment of this area, needles with a diameter of 0.2 mm are inserted at a depth of 2 cm [4].

We present the effects of acupuncture treatment on the upper limb on a case of occupational dystonia of the upper limb that we have experienced. The patient was a cook who frequently held his left hand, which was thought to have caused dystonia in the left upper limb (Case 4). At the time of initial acupuncture treatment, he had difficulty in opening his left hand. After 15 minutes of acupuncture treatment to the upper-limb area, the patient's left hand opening movement improved (**Figure 5**).

After acupuncture treatment in the upper-limb area, he can smoothly open his fingers.

Before acupuncture

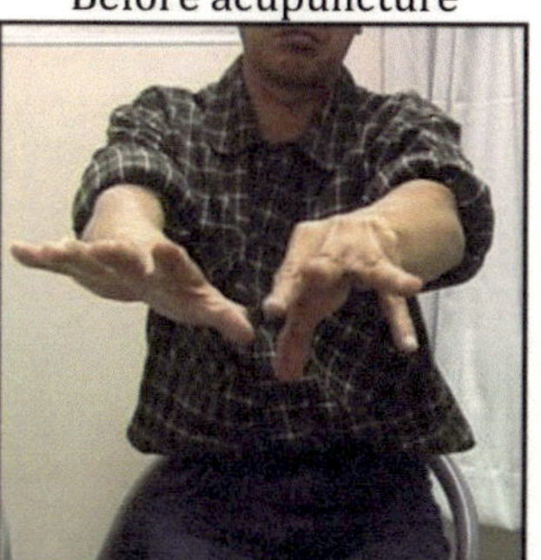

15 minutes after acupuncture

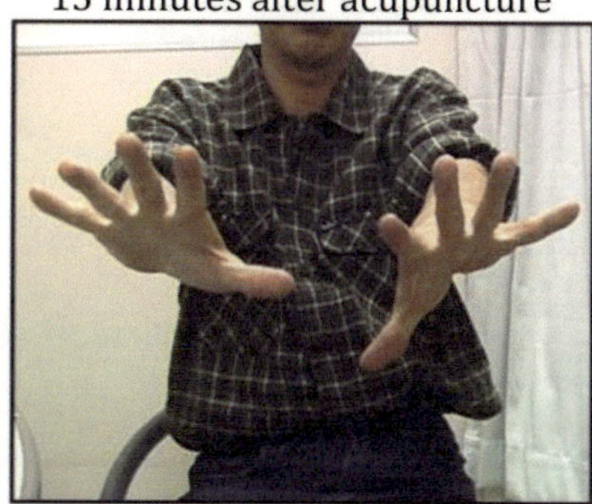

Figure 5.
Hand opening and closing movements before and after initial acupuncture treatment.

5. Mechanisms of acupuncture effects

We consider the mechanism of acupuncture's effect on dystonia to be as follows: First, cutaneous stimulation by acupuncture needles becomes a painful stimulus that ascends the lateral spinal thalamic tract, synapses in the thalamus, and projects to the somatosensory cortex as tertiary neurons. The inhibitory effects in the somatosensory and motor cortices then work at the cortical level to inhibit the descending pyramidal tract and α-motor neurons, resulting in relaxation of muscle tone.

The other is that a similar stimulus may have caused inhibition of extrapyramidal impulses at the thalamic and cortical levels, resulting in a reduction in muscle tone due to inhibition of γ-motor neurons.

6. Conclusion

We introduced our acupuncture treatment for cervical dystonia and upper extremity dystonia. The advantages of acupuncture include its ability to treat both hypertonia and hypotonia, the muscle tone abnormalities of dystonia; its ability to treat secondary disorders such as muscle shortening and skin shortening; and the fact that it rarely causes side effects. However, consistent improvement of symptoms requires long-term treatment; it is important to accumulate improvement after each treatment and to continue treatment patiently, paying attention to changes in the patient's symptoms.

Author details

Makiko Tani* and Toshiaki Suzuki
Graduate School, Kansai University of Health Sciences, Osaka, Japan

*Address all correspondence to: tani@kansai.ac.jp

References

[1] Steeves TD, Day L, Dykeman J, et al. The prevalence of primary dystonia: A systematic review and meta-analysis. Movement Disorders. 2012;**27**:1789-1796

[2] Suzuki T, Tani M, Nabeta R, Wakayama I, Yase Y. Évaluation clinique et électromyographique de l'effect de l'acpuncture sur les patients souffrants de torticolis spasmodique (In French). MÉRIDIENS. 2000;**115**(2):17-26

[3] Tani M, Suzuki T, Wakayama I, et al. Acupuncture for cervical dystonia. The Journal of Kampo, Acupuncture and Integrative Medicine (KAIM). 2006;**1**:13-18

[4] Tani M, Suzuki T, Wakayama I, Yoshida S. How do you treat dystonic movements in the upper extremity in your practice? Medical Acupuncture. 2017;**29**:29-25. DOI: 10.1089/acu.2017.29065.cpl

[5] World Health Organization/WHO Western Pacific Region Office. WHO Standard Acupuncture Point Locations in the Western Pacific Region. Switzerland: World Health Organization; 2008

[6] Hallett M. Is dystonia a sensory disorder? Annals of Neurology. 1995;**38**(2):139-140. DOI: 10.1002/ana.410380203